D0153215

Debating Modern Medical Technologies

Debating Modern Medical Technologies

The Politics of Safety, Effectiveness, and Patient Access

Karen J. Maschke and Michael K. Gusmano

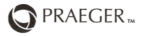 PRAEGER™

An Imprint of ABC-CLIO, LLC

Santa Barbara, California • Denver, Colorado

Library of Congress Cataloging-in-Publication Data

Names: Maschke, Karen J., author. | Gusmano, Michael K., author.
Title: Debating modern medical technologies : the politics of safety, effectiveness, and patient access / Karen J. Maschke and Michael K. Gusmano.
Description: Santa Barbara, California : ABC-CLIO, LLC, [2018] | Includes bibliographical references and index.
Identifiers: LCCN 2018036668 (print) | LCCN 2018036936 (ebook) | ISBN 9781440861901 (ebook) | ISBN 9781440861895 (set : alk. paper)
Subjects: LCSH: Medical technology—Political aspects. | Medical technology—Safety measures. | Medical technology—Social aspects.
Classification: LCC R855.3 (ebook) | LCC R855.3 .M3774 2018 (print) | DDC 610.28/9—dc23
LC record available at https://lccn.loc.gov/2018036668

ISBN: 978-1-4408-6189-5 (print)
      978-1-4408-6190-1 (ebook)

22 21 20 19 18   1 2 3 4 5

This book is also available as an eBook.

Praeger
An Imprint of ABC-CLIO, LLC

ABC-CLIO, LLC
130 Cremona Drive, P.O. Box 1911
Santa Barbara, California 93116-1911
www.abc-clio.com

This book is printed on acid-free paper ∞
Manufactured in the United States of America

Contents

Acknowledgments

We would like to thank the Hastings Center for its generous support of our work. We received Daniel Callahan and Willard Gaylin Fund Awards from the Hastings Center to support our writing. Along with our thanks to colleagues at the Hastings Center, we would like to thank the faculty at Rutgers University and colleagues at the Health Politics and Policy Section of the American Political Science Association who provided helpful feedback on the work. The book is much stronger, thanks to the feedback we received, and we alone are responsible for any remaining errors.

CHAPTER ONE

Evidence, Politics, and Medical Care Technology

> Facts do not find their way into the world in which our beliefs reside;
> they did not produce our beliefs, they do not destroy them; they may
> inflict on them the most constant refutations without weakening them,
> and an avalanche of afflictions or ailments succeeding one another
> without interruption in a family will not make it doubt the goodness of
> its God or the talent of its doctor.
>
> —Marcel Proust, *Swann's Way*[1]

Debates over health care reform in the United States often focus on the need
to expand access to medical care services by expanding health insurance and
reducing the out-of-pocket costs faced by patients and their families. Appropriate medical care can alleviate suffering, extend life, and, for some patients,
cure disease. Investments in biological and clinical research have produced
improvements in therapy that have significantly reduced premature death
due to many diseases. Even though there is no question that medical care
can provide enormous benefits, there is growing concern that patients often
receive diagnostic, preventive, and therapeutic medical technologies for
which there is limited or conflicting evidence.[2] According to some estimates,
"less than half of medical care in the United States is based on or supported
by evidence about its effectiveness, often resulting in care that is inappropriate and unnecessary."[3] Thus, slogans like "evidence-based medicine" not-
withstanding, the reality of health care in the United States is that some
patients receive treatments and diagnostic tests that offer little or no benefit,
some fail to receive interventions that may be highly beneficial, and some

may be harmed by side effects of drugs or by unnecessary diagnostic tests and procedures that are not outweighed by improved medical outcomes, if any.[4]

This book draws on ideas from science and technology studies that raise important questions about the nature of science as well as disputes about evidence and political science to examine what values and interests about government regulation, cost-effectiveness, risks and benefits to patients and society, and technological innovation shape policy debates and initiatives regarding evidence and access to new medical technologies.[5] We build on the work of scholars who examine epistemological issues concerning technology assessment and evidence-based medicine, including those who critique claims that rigorous evidence of safety and effectiveness should be based on data from randomized controlled trials (RCT)[6] as well as those who analyze the regulatory, sociopolitical, and economic factors that play a role in how evidence disputes are framed.[7] The book's conceptual framework also draws from a long tradition of political science theories about the policy process to better understand how ideas, interests, and institutions are shaping policy decisions regarding market entry and payer coverage for medical technologies and the meaning and implementation of evidence-based medicine.[8]

Our framework assumes that ideas about science and government matter a great deal. There are serious disagreements among scientists, clinicians, insurance executives, patient advocates, and elected officials about what counts as evidence when evaluating medical technology. There are also disagreements about the extent to which government regulations and market mechanisms should be used to make decisions about what technologies to use and how to pay for them. But while we recognize the importance of intellectual disputes over how to make decisions about medical technologies, we place the role of ideas in the context of political and economic opportunities and constraints. Disputes about evidence standards include legitimate scientific disagreement about the type and amount of evidence needed to make claims about a medical technology's safety and effectiveness. In recent years, however, "evidence disputes" have also been pulled into the universe of "alternative facts." The "war on science"[9] has expanded to include debates about the evaluation of medical technologies and claims by those who are skeptical of science and question the authority of experts to render judgments about what does and does not work in medical care.[10]

Yet, while disagreements about science are important, the intersection of values, interests, politics, and economics frame and shape disputes about evidence, influence policy initiatives about evidence standards, and play a role in government agency decision making regarding the clinical use of and payment for new medical technologies. Policy makers often have difficulty challenging and resisting powerful stakeholders' claims that using less rigorous, less systematic, and less transparent evidentiary standards for assessing the safety and effectiveness of medical technologies will not result in harm to patients, despite clear historical examples that this is not the case.[11]

We illustrate how competing ideas about science, interest groups, and political ideology—by which we mean ideas about the role of government in society—frame debates about the potential benefits and harms of medical technologies. One facet of these debates involves ideas about what counts as good medical science—or what philosophers call the "epistemology" of evidence.[12] How much and what kind of evidence of safety and effectiveness is needed before the U.S. Food and Drug Administration (FDA) should permit a drug or device company to market its product for clinical use? Are RCTs always necessary to obtain safety and effectiveness evidence, or can sufficient evidence of effectiveness be obtained from other sources, such as observational studies, disease registries, and patient self-reports? Should evidentiary standards for patient access to medical technologies be the same for preventive, diagnostic, or treatment purposes and for drugs and medical devices? Should public and private health insurers automatically pay for a drug or device the FDA approved? Is it acceptable for public or private payers to include information about cost-effectiveness in their decisions about coverage, or does such analysis reflect inappropriate assumptions about the public's "willingness to pay" for such technologies?[13] Even if payers use an economic evaluation of medical technologies and determine that they are cost-effective, how should policy makers balance demands for greater spending on medical technology with demands to address other important social needs? Can evidence about a drug's cost-effectiveness help to answer these questions? What if patients want access to drugs and devices that the FDA has not approved, and their physician wants to provide the interventions to them?

These debates involve not only questions about appropriate scientific method but also disagreements about who gets to decide whether there is enough evidence that a medical technology's benefits outweigh its risks or whether its benefits are "worth" the cost. As with debates about national health insurance, opponents of government regulation often frame efforts to limit the use of medical technologies as an effort to inappropriately limit physician autonomy or interfere with the doctor-patient relationship. In the 1940s, the American Medical Association (AMA) began a nearly $5 million campaign to defeat national health insurance.[14] They hired the public relations firm of Whitaker and Baxter and provided them with a $1.6 million budget for 1949 alone.[15] Whitaker and Baxter made effective use of the special social role played by doctors and the emotional ties that they had with their patients. In their now infamous poster, Whitaker and Baxter displayed a reproduction of Sir Luke Fildes's painting of a doctor at the bedside of a sick child. Underneath the picture the poster read:

> Voluntary Health Insurance—The American Way—WILL KEEP POLITICS OUT OF THIS PICTURE! When the life—or health of a loved one is at stake, hope lies in the devoted service of your Doctor. Would you change this picture? Compulsory health insurance is political medicine. It would bring a third party—a politician—between you and your Doctor. It would bind up your family's health in red tape. It would result in heavy payroll taxes—and inferior medical care for you and your family. Don't let that happen here! You have a right to prepaid medical care—of your own choice. Ask your Doctor, or your insurance man about budget-basis health protection.[16]

This fear of government interference resurfaces frequently in debates about U.S. health policy. Calls for allowing government to regulate the price of drugs, for example, are frequently met with the claim that this will suppress innovation and destroy jobs. In response to concerns that President Obama's administration would try to negotiate the price of medications purchased by the Medicare program, David Williams, the president of the Taxpayers Protection Alliance, wrote that "giving federal agencies the power to negotiate drug prices is a sure fire way of stifling innovation and taking away incentives for the development of new medicines."[17] In 2012, the *Wall Street Journal* published an article indicating that FDA regulations would drive drug companies out of the country and lead to a "mass exodus" of jobs to countries with less onerous regulatory requirements.[18] The idea that government regulation of the drug industry drives up prices, drives out industry, and fails to advance the public interest is frequently invoked by free-market advocates.[19] In contrast, others argue that Congress has made it much easier for the FDA to bring drugs to market and that it has done little, if anything, to regulate prices.[20]

What role should government agencies play in determining the evidentiary standards for market entry and patients' access to medical technologies? What role should the companies that develop these technologies have in this decision-making process? Should decisions about whether and under what circumstances patients can use medical technologies be left to patients and their physicians? These questions suggest that ideas and values matter. Political fights about health technology assessment and the meaning and implementation of evidence-based medicine reflect values about patient choice, physician autonomy, and government intervention in medicine and technology assessment. It is important to investigate what values shape how a medical technology's risks and benefits are framed and the evidentiary approaches to evaluating those risks and benefits.[21]

Of course, it is also important to remember that there is a lot of money at stake. Health economist Uwe Reinhardt famously remarked that "every dollar of health care spending is a dollar of income,"[22] and the implications of this reality are evident in the cases we examine. In 2016, *Forbes* magazine reported that medical technology was projected to be the most profitable sector, "with a 21.6% net profit margin."[23] In recent years, generic drug companies have experienced profit margins of just over 5 percent, but the major drug companies have profit margins that are over 18 percent.[24] Along with pharmaceutical industry profits, the U.S. Government Accountability Office found that, between 2005 and 2014, medical device companies experienced a 44 percent increase in profits, even though the Patient Protection and Affordable Care Act of 2010 (ACA) imposed new taxes on such devices.[25] Whenever there is a push to regulate medical care technology, organizations that profit from these technologies mobilize to shape, if not stop, this regulation. When doing so, they often reframe the political debate to emphasize the degree to which policy choices are about economic development and jobs. From this perspective, public and private spending on medical technologies is not a disaster; it improves health directly by providing treatments for illness and indirectly because it is a growth industry that provides jobs.

The idea that companies that produce medical technologies would push for their use is not surprising, but our cases remind us that other stakeholders, including patient advocacy groups, often join with pharmaceutical and biotechnology companies to push for faster adoption and broader use of medical technologies. This does not imply that patient advocates and other consumer groups are always in favor of faster FDA approval of technologies or of evidence from sources other than RCTs, but as political scientist David Truman reminded us in the 1950s, politics often involves complex and surprising coalitions of groups with overlapping interests.[26] In short, political disputes regarding the development, market entry, and payer coverage of medical technologies are shaped by the broader political economy in which they take place.[27]

Powerful organizations are pushing for the adoption of nontraditional research designs and methods of analysis to speed market approval for new medical technologies tested in human clinical trials and to relax evidentiary standards for assessing the safety and effectiveness of those technologies.[28] These groups include pharmaceutical companies and device manufacturers as well as an array of advocacy groups. Although some patient advocacy groups have been accused of being fronts for pharmaceutical companies, many are not. Various "coalitions of interest" are also coalescing in support of initiatives to give some patients greater access to medical technologies being tested in clinical trials that still have an incomplete evidence base from research studies about their therapeutic efficacy and side effects.[29] These perspectives were incorporated into the 21st Century Cures Act (hereinafter Cures Act) approved by Congress in December 2016.[30] For example, the Cures Act allows the FDA to rely on "data summaries," rather than phase III clinical trials, to support the approval of drugs for new indications, and it permits pharmaceutical companies to promote off-label uses of their products to insurance companies. The Cures Act also incorporates a broad definition of "breakthrough" medical devices that will expand and speed up the FDA's approval process for devices for patients with life-limiting and debilitating diseases or conditions for which there are limited alternative treatments. President Donald Trump has joined the call for reducing regulation and getting faster FDA approval for new medical technologies. When the president met with leaders of the pharmaceutical industry at the White House in January 2017, he said, "We're going to be cutting regulations at a level nobody's ever seen before. . . . You're going to get your products—either approved or not approved—but it's going to be a quick process."[31]

At the same time, public and private payers are more resistant to providing coverage for new, expensive medical technologies, even though many patient advocates believe that such technologies may be highly effective. In 2015, for example, the FDA approved new cholesterol-lowering drugs called PCSK9 inhibitors that decrease low-density lipoprotein cholesterol levels—but they are quite expensive, and insurance companies frequently refuse to cover them.[32] Physicians and patient advocacy groups often claim that decisions of this sort are an effort to save money even though the new drugs are more effective than those already in use. In response, insurers claim that for many new, expensive drugs, particularly those for rare diseases, "there is no data pool, no pharmacoeconomics analysis, and it is becoming more and more of an issue."[33]

This means that the fight over medical technology is not simply a story of powerful economic interests versus the public interest—it is often a fight among competing interests about the meaning of the public interest. The "powerful interest group model" of the policy process is familiar to students of politics and argues that economic forces often dominate considerations of the evidence when payers make coverage decisions.[34] For most of the modern era, political science viewed public policies as the results of demands placed on the political system from outside sources.[35] Explanations of public policy offered by political scientists until the 1980s tended to stress the importance of social forces, ignoring the important role played by political and economic institutions in structuring social choices.[36] The past three decades have witnessed a movement to reverse this trend.[37] State-centered theorists have offered what Peter Hall calls a "corrective to the pluralist emphases on the societal sources of policy" by arguing that the state plays an independent role in shaping public policy.[38] We draw on these institutional theories and discuss how values and interests operate within the context of political institutions. Through our case studies, we illustrate how courts, lawmakers, regulatory agencies, and political parties influence the rules of the game that govern evidentiary standards for evaluating the safety and effectiveness of medical technologies and the coverage decisions of public and private insurers.

Policy debates about evidentiary standards for assessing the safety and effectiveness of medical technologies are caught up in the maelstrom of partisan electoral politics, where short-term responses to complex problems have become the norm. Partisan differences about the role of government often frame the nature of these debates. This is not new, but arguments about what counts as appropriate evidence and which institutions should be allowed to make such decisions have intensified and reflect the widening gap between Democrats and Republicans in Congress about the appropriate role of government in regulating the economy, including medical technologies. When debates about medical technologies take place during broader debates about the government's role in financing health care, the partisan framing of this issue becomes especially acute. In two of the cases we present in this book—the debate over the use of mammography screening and the FDA's decision to limit the use of Avastin, a cancer drug—it is almost impossible to separate the political debate over medical technology from the debate over the ACA. In all our cases, however, partisan disagreements are just beneath the surface of the debate.

To better understand how these forces shape evidence disputes and policy making, this book draws on five case studies. The first two focus on debates about the value of diagnostic technologies. One of the diagnostic technologies we examine—mammography screening—has been around for years, and fights about its use involve the interpretation of evidence accumulated over decades. The second technology—positron emission tomography (PET) scans to measure amyloid-beta plaque in the living brain—is a more recent fight that involves questions about what kind of evidence about therapeutic benefits health insurers want to see before they are willing to pay for medical technologies.

The mammography case illustrates the concern about overdiagnosis and explores the debate about the value of mammography screening. In 2009, the U.S. Preventive Services Task Force (USPSTF) issued a recommendation against routine mammography screening for women under the age of 40 unless they were in a high-risk category. The recommendation, which was issued in the midst of the debate over the proposed ACA, created a political firestorm. In response, Congress incorporated language into the final version of the ACA instructing insurers, providers, and patients to ignore the USPSTF recommendations. But this case is not only about partisan disagreements about the regulation of clinical care; it is also a story about the power of certain patient advocacy groups and their ability to influence the perceptions of the public and policy makers about how to respond to a disease. Through social marketing campaigns, several powerful breast cancer advocacy groups have spent years convincing the public that mammography screening saves lives and attacks on coverage of mammography screening are attacks on women's health. A large body of scientific evidence that casts doubt on the value of mammography screening was insufficient to counter the influence of partisan and interest group forces.

The second case explores the decision by the Centers for Medicare and Medicaid Services (CMS) not to pay for certain Medicare beneficiaries to undergo a PET scan designed to detect the presence of amyloid-beta plaque in the living brain. Amyloid-beta plaque is correlated with Alzheimer's disease, but whether there is a causal relationship between this plaque and Alzheimer's disease is still in dispute. Until recently, a definitive diagnosis of Alzheimer's disease was only possible after identifying amyloid plaque in a patient's brain at autopsy. In 2010, Lilly USA received FDA approval for a contrast dye that, when used in conjunction with a PET scan, could detect amyloid plaque in the living brain. Despite FDA approval, CMS refused to pay for this test under the Medicare program because it concluded that it would not change the course of treatment or result in better patient outcomes. This represented a break from precedent because Medicare has usually agreed to pay for technologies approved by the FDA. The Medicare decision in this case remains an outlier, but it will be important to track whether program officials raise similar questions about other new technologies. CMS officials under the Trump administration may be less inclined to use the authority of government to challenge the value of medical technologies developed by the private sector, but the budget pressures faced by Medicare may be even greater as the administration attempts to limit government spending on health and social services.

The third case explores another controversy about payer coverage—this time about the criteria for deciding whether to pay for expensive new treatments for hepatitis C. Since 2013, the FDA has approved a number of antiviral drugs for hepatitis C capable of eliminating detectable levels of the virus for many patients. Although prices have decreased in recent years, the price of all these new drugs is still extremely high, initially costing nearly $100,000 per treatment. In response to the price, both public and private insurers have sought to limit the availability of these drugs. One strategy that insurers adopted was to limit coverage for these drugs to patients who have already experienced liver damage as a result of their hepatitis C infection, arguing that the treatment ought to go to those in greatest need and that there is insufficient evidence from the initial clinical trials to justify the use of these treatments in people with an early diagnosis. In response, a number of patients filed lawsuits against several insurance companies and state Medicaid programs, arguing there is sufficient evidence about the effectiveness of these drugs among those with an early diagnosis, and thus public and private insurers should not be allowed to restrict access to drugs that physicians decide their patients need. In 2014, the Patient Centered Outcomes Research Institute (PCORI) decided to address this controversy. PCORI held a stakeholder meeting at which they decided to fund research that would establish the effectiveness of providing treatment to patients recently diagnosed with hepatitis C but before they have developed liver damage, but after stakeholders objected, PCORI reversed its decision and decided not to pursue this research. This case clearly illustrates how debates about research and evidence become intimately linked with ideological ideas about the role of government and interests. This debate centers on disagreements about how to assess the value of new therapies, but it is also a case about the political and economic consequences of failing to negotiate prices in the health care system. This failure, coupled with efforts to reduce total health care spending, sets up disputes among providers, patients, and payers about how to cope with the high cost of care.

The last two cases involve the evidentiary standards for FDA market approval of new medical technologies—and withdrawing such approval after patients have used them to treat their disease. In 2010, the FDA decided to revoke its approval of bevacizumab (Avastin), a drug to treat metastatic breast cancer. This case raises important questions about the evidence standards that should be used under the agency's accelerated approval pathway. In response to demands from Congress, patient advocates, and industry, the FDA has created mechanisms that allow drugs to reach the market faster. The Cures Act calls for further increasing the speed with which some treatments are allowed to go to market. The Avastin case raises questions about how to balance demands for faster access with concerns about safety and effectiveness and about the FDA's willingness to require or recommend market withdrawal when postapproval studies show a drug has limited effectiveness or that serious side effects outweigh its therapeutic benefit. It also highlights the potential consequences of the failure to demand the timely completion of postmarketing studies by drug companies. The questions the Avastin case raised will likely arise again as the FDA implements provisions of the Cures Act that provide an expedited pathway for the development and review of stem cell and other regenerative medicine interventions.

The final case focuses on debates about the FDA's regulatory authority over stem cell and other regenerative medicine interventions and the evidentiary requirements for market entry of those interventions. Unlike medical drugs, these types of interventions involve the use—separately or in combination—of human cells, genes, and tissues. Some patients, physicians, and others claim that some stem cell interventions fall outside the FDA's regulatory purview and thus should not be subject to the agency's premarket approval requirements, including obtaining safety and effectiveness data from RCTs.[39] One dimension of the stem cell dispute is about obtaining safety and effectiveness evidence through a regulatory versus a "medical innovation" pathway.[40] The FDA recently announced that it is developing a more consistent regulatory framework governing stem cell and other regenerative medicine interventions, and the Cures Act contains provisions for an expedited development and review pathway for the stem cell interventions the FDA regulates. The Cures Act and other federal and state policy initiatives draw attention to whether and the extent to which values about risks and benefits of new medical technologies and global political economy pressures play a role in policy initiatives regarding access to stem cell and other regenerative medicine interventions.

The case studies in this book were selected for several reasons. All these cases have elements of controversy about the evidentiary standards government agencies use to evaluate the effectiveness or the value of new medical technologies. Much of the debate in the United States about health technology assessment and the meaning and implementation of evidence-based medicine is about the clinical context in which physicians decide what diagnostic, preventive, and treatment interventions to use in the face of little or conflicting evidence about safety and effectiveness.[41] By focusing primarily, though not exclusively, on the federal regulatory and payer contexts, this book provides an opportunity to investigate the values, interests, and assumptions that various stakeholders bring to these contexts about evidence standards and patient access to new medical technologies.

The in-depth analysis of these cases also presents an opportunity to consider whether and how varying risks and benefits; physician and patient users; and scientific, clinical, and regulatory goals across the technologies examined may influence the discourse about evidentiary standards, patient access, and policy initiatives to encourage the diffusion of these new medical technologies into the clinic. We examine how the framing of scientific paradigms about the technologies influences how various stakeholders approach their assessment.[42]

To set the context for the case study discussions, chapter 2 provides a brief history of the politics of health technology assessment in the United States. Until the late 1960s, federal policy makers paid relatively little attention to the issues of cost and quality in medical care. For example, enhancing access to mainstream health care was the principle concern of the architects of the Medicare program.[43] Following the program's enactment in 1965, Congress mandated quality assurance programs for Medicare beneficiaries,[44] but very little emphasis was placed on improving the quality or efficiency of health care delivery in the United States.[45] To the contrary, the noninterference clause of Title XVIII of the Social Security Act, which is the initial authorizing legislation for the Medicare program, explicitly sought to limit the ability of the government to regulate medical providers. It reads:

> Nothing in this title shall be construed to authorize any Federal officer or employee to exercise any supervision or control over the practice of medicine or the manner in which medical services are provided . . . or to exercise any supervision or control over the administration or operation of any . . . institution, agency, or person [providing health care services].[46]

The Medicare law did set up minimal quality standards for hospitals that wanted to participate in the program. Any hospital that wanted to participate had to be certified by the Joint Commission on the Accreditation of Hospitals—now called the Joint Commission.[47] Joint Commission's accreditation process draws on a structure (who provides care and where), process (how care is provided), and outcomes approach to the measurement of quality that Avedis Donabedian advocated for in his seminal 1966 article, "Evaluating the Quality of Medicare Care."[48] Since the early 1990s, Joint Commission has also drawn on theories of continuous quality improvement developed by W. Edwards Deming, Walter A. Shewhart, and Joseph M. Juran.[49] The only quality standard for physicians was the requirement that services had to be "medically necessary."

There were two reasons for the initial lack of emphasis on quality. First, legislators were concerned about the willingness of physicians to participate in the Medicare program. Supporters of Medicare within Congress feared that if they attempted to place more stringent requirements on providers, the legislation creating the program might not pass Congress at all. As with the decision to pay physicians' "usual and customary fees" as long as they were "reasonable" and to allow physicians to charge patients more than the government was willing to reimburse, the decision not to interfere with the practice of medicine by regulating quality was shaped by the fear that physicians would act on their frequently repeated threat and refuse to participate in the Medicare program.[50]

Second, most people assumed that expanding access to the mainstream health care system would be enough to improve the quality of care received by Medicare beneficiaries. Even after decades of evidence that the U.S. health care system suffers from significant quality problems, the idea that the United States has the "best health care system in the world" still resonates with political leaders.[51] When voicing opposition to the ACA in 2011 after the Republicans took control of the U.S. House of Representatives, Speaker-elect John Boehner argued that it would "ruin the best health care system in the world."[52] In March 2017, when calling on Republican members of Congress to "repeal and replace" the ACA, Vice President Mike Pence claimed, "We're going to make the best healthcare system in the world even better."[53]

Despite the frequently repeated refrain about the high quality of the U.S. health care system, concerns about its cost—and about whether its high price is generating good value—have produced growing concerns about its performance. After the adoption of Medicare and Medicaid in 1965, however, the cost of health care became a major focus of policy makers, and, by the 1970s, concerns about quality began to emerge as well. A number of studies raised questions about the value of many medical technologies and argued that variations in the use of technology—and spending on it—were not explained by differences in need or outcome. This led policy makers and private insurance companies to question the value of medical technologies and adopt more aggressive efforts to assess their diagnostic, preventive, and therapeutic benefits, efforts that have frequently met with resistance. The fight between those who emphasize the need for better evidence about the value of medical technologies and those who wish to expand their availability to patients are reflected in each of the cases we present in this book and involve a complex interplay of ideas about science, politics, and material interests.

Evolving Public- and Private-Payer Approaches to Evidence and Health Technology Assessment

Researchers and the media frequently document concerns about the quality of health care. Studies have found that patients receive only about 50 percent of recommended preventive, acute, and chronic care.[1] Others have documented preventable medical errors associated with surgeries and preventable hospital-acquired infections.[2] And along with stories about the remarkable gains associated with medical technologies,[3] there are also stories about patients who are harmed by these technologies.[4]

Until the end of the 1960s, health policy debates in the United States focused primarily on the extent to which the federal government should guarantee access to health care for its citizens through some type of public-payer health insurance system. Neither the cost nor the quality of the health care system were major concerns for policy makers.[5] After creating the Medicare program in 1965 to provide health insurance for United States' seniors, Congress mandated quality assurance programs for Medicare beneficiaries,[6] but very little emphasis was placed on improving the efficiency of health care delivery in the United States.[7] Policy makers assumed that if the government could help people overcome financial barriers to getting health care by providing insurance coverage for them, they "would enjoy the best in health care that the nation could offer, and quality would be a 'nonissue.'"[8] Even after decades of evidence that the U.S. health care system suffers from significant quality problems, the idea that the United States has the "best health care system in the world" still resonates with members of Congress.[9]

Other than setting minimal quality standards for hospitals, the initial policy focused on Medicare beneficiaries' enrollment and access to entitled benefits. The lack of emphasis on quality was consistent with Medicare's deference to hospitals and physicians at the start of the program.[10,11] The main administrative elements of the program were carried out by regional insurance companies (Part A fiscal intermediaries and Part B carriers—usually the state's Blue Cross/Blue Shield plans). Federal policy makers at the Social Security Administration, which had responsibility for the Medicare and Medicaid programs until the establishment of the Health Care Financing Administration (HCFA) in 1977, assumed that in the process of paying claims under the rubric of "medically necessary" and "usual, customary, and reasonable" services, these insurance companies were, in effect, screening for quality.[12] Once the FDA approved a medical technology for use, the Medicare program typically allowed it to become part of the benefit package and allowed medical professionals to determine whether it was appropriate for their Medicare patients and private health insurers to decide whether they would pay for it.

Yet along with private payers, the Medicare program did not always agree to pay for a medical technology the FDA approved. Public and private payers also often refused to pay for technologies, tests, and procedures for which FDA approval was not required, and for "off-label" use of a technology, i.e., for a diagnostic or therapeutic use that is different from the specific purpose the FDA approved for market entry. As we discuss in the following sections, central to the evolving health policy initiatives and payer coverage policies that shifted attention to quality and value was the issue of evidence about the effectiveness of medical technologies: do they actually work as intended for the patients who will use them?

Evidence and the Influence of Scientific Medicine

The origins of scientific medicine, with an emphasis on controlled experiments, go back to the 16th century and the influence of the Enlightenment on medicine.[13] Over the next five centuries, clinical researchers experimented with new methods for conducting research to determine the safety and effectiveness of medical technologies. In 1948, the British Medical Research Council used an RCT to evaluate the drug streptomycin for the treatment of tuberculosis.[14] While there is an ongoing debate about alternative methods for evaluating whether medical technologies are safe and effective, RCTs have continued to be viewed by many as the gold standard for doing so,[15] and the FDA has traditionally relied heavily on evidence from RCTs in determining whether to grant market approval for its regulatory decisions. However, as we discuss in chapters six and seven, the agency has come under increasing pressure from multiple stakeholders—including conservative interest groups and some members of Congress—to evaluate drugs for market entry on the basis of evidence from sources other than RCTs.

In 1889, Baltimore banker and philanthropist Johns Hopkins, who wanted to promote medical education reform of the kind taking place in Europe, left instructions in his will for the establishment of a hospital and medical school. Johns Hopkins was not the first university to affiliate a teaching hospital with a medical school, but Hopkins moved more aggressively in this direction and recruited several young clinicians who were familiar with trends in Europe. For example, Dr. William Osler, professor of medicine, established bedside teaching and the training of third- and fourth-year medical students on the hospital wards and introduced the German residency system, which established postmedical school training in hospitals for young physicians.[16]

Johns Hopkins University revolutionized the teaching of medicine in the United States, and this approach was valorized by Abraham Flexner from the Carnegie Foundation for the Advancement of Teaching who, in 1910, published a report on medical education in the United States based on visits to all 155 medical schools in the country at that time.[17] Flexner criticized medical education for its lack of focus on science and its poor quality. His report had a transformative effect on medical education and the profession. The Flexner report emphasized the need for medical schools to adopt "formal analytic reasoning" as the basis for training physicians.[18] The emphasis on evidence-based medicine, including the use of RCTs, continued to grow throughout the 20th century.[19]

Just a few years before the Flexner report, Congress adopted and President Theodore Roosevelt signed into law the Food and Drugs Act of 1906. After decades of proposals to regulate the food industry in the United States, accounts by so-called muckraking writers, including Upton Sinclair, whose book *The Jungle* documented the conditions of the meatpacking industry, helped lead to the adoption of the new law. It prohibited interstate commerce in misbranded and adulterated foods, drinks, and drugs. Under the 1906 act, the federal government was authorized to regulate product labeling rather than premarket approval, and the primary focus was on food. The act was expanded by Congress several times and, in 1938, Congress adopted the U.S. Food, Drug, and Cosmetic Act (FDCA) and gave the FDA authority to require that pharmaceutical products the agency regulated had to obtain approval from the agency before market entry. This represented a major shift in policy and expansion of government authority over what medical technologies entered the market. Under this system, drug manufacturers are required to apply for market approval by providing data to the FDA of animal and human testing. The data submitted to the FDA must show "substantial evidence" of effectiveness. This required animal studies first, followed by several phases of human studies. The first phase tests for safety with a small number (20 to 100) of healthy volunteers and/or people with the disease. The second phase investigates efficacy with a larger sample (usually several hundred people) with the disease. The third phase involves a much larger sample (often in the thousands) to conduct further tests of efficacy and side effects. Phase four involves the postmarketing surveillance of drugs.

Often prompted and sometimes mandated by Congress, the FDA has developed several pathways to expedite the review and approval of new drugs and biologics for serious conditions, but the basic approach the FDCA established requiring FDA market approval on the basis of evidence of safety and effectiveness from human clinical trials remains in place to this day. The role of the FDA in establishing evidentiary standards for market entry of medical technologies and its strong public reputation,[20] coupled with the medical profession's role in developing the standards for scientific medicine, help to explain the lack of focus on quality and evidence when Medicare and Medicaid were adopted in 1965. Once the cost of health care reached the public policy agenda, however, the situation changed dramatically.

From Cost Crisis to Value for Money

By the end of the 1960s, the health policy agenda in the United States shifted dramatically. In 1969, greater awareness among policy makers, the media, and the public about the escalation of health care costs led President Nixon to declare that the U.S. health care system was facing a "massive crisis in this area."[21] In that same year, the financial magazines *Business Week* and *Fortune* ran stories that described a system "on the brink of chaos."[22] Two changes in the health care system led to this sudden, widespread of concern about how much the government and private health insurers were spending and what they were buying.

One change was the continual increase in health care spending as a percentage of gross national product (GNP). Although this increase emerged decades before the creation of the Medicare and Medicaid programs in 1965, it became much more pronounced in the years following their implementation. This was due in part to an increase in demand, but primarily due to increases in the cost of care and development of new technologies. Health costs rose by 13 percent as a proportion of GNP in the five years before these programs were enacted. They rose by 20 percent in the five years following their enactment.[23]

Second, and perhaps more importantly, the federal government began paying a much larger share of the nation's health care bill. The most dramatic change in our health care system between 1960 and 1970 was the percentage of our health care expenditures paid for by the federal government. State and local health spending remained relatively stable between 1960 and 1970, but federal health spending as a percentage of total government spending nearly tripled during this time period.

The budget implications of the federal government's decision to create two new public health insurance programs, Medicare and Medicaid, without any attempt to restructure the way health care was financed quickly became apparent to elected officials, businesspeople, journalists, and the general public. Until the federal government took responsibility for a large percentage of health care costs, the public debate had focused almost exclusively on whether and how the government should expand access to medical care by paying for some of the costs. Since the adoption of Medicare, the debate over health care has centered much of its attention on how to contain costs, although few public policies in the United States represent serious efforts to actually reduce them.[24]

The government's new role as health care insurer not only saw a dramatic increase in the amount of attention given to health care generally, it changed the focus of the government's inquiry and its assessment of the problem. By 1970, both liberal and conservative critics of the system began to point the finger at health care providers as the cause of the health care system's problems and the major obstacle to its reform.[25] Initial attempts to confront the issue of rising health care costs, however, continued the pattern of deference to providers.

On top of the budgetary pressures caused by the growth in Medicare and Medicaid spending, there was growing skepticism about the quality of the medical technologies the programs' beneficiaries were using, as well as their necessity. Paul Starr argued that the public's willingness to question the wisdom of physicians who recommended or prescribed various technologies blossomed to the point that the "nineteenth century doctrine of therapeutic nihilism—that drugs and therapies were useless—was revived in a new form."[26] These attacks came from both ends of the political spectrum and were given voice by books such as *Doing Better and Feeling Worse* by Aaron Wildavsky and *Medical Nemesis* by Ivan Illich.[27] In more recent years, Daniel Callahan has been a leading critic of the medical care system, arguing that it has become obsessed with the goal of life extension and the continual pursuit of new, expensive medical technologies, regardless of whether they work for their intended purpose or work better than those already available.[28]

The main point of these medical care critics was that environmental, social, and behavioral factors had a greater impact on individual health than medical care.[29] As Starr points out, the irony of this attack on medical care was that it came about at a time when the country was making extraordinary strides against death and disease.[30] Nevertheless, these concerns worked to reinforce the idea that we were wasting money on health care and that we needed to find a way to rein in our health care spending. Decades later, critics made similar claims during the debate over the Clinton and Obama administration health care proposals.[31]

Most health economists argue that there is no "right" amount of money to spend on health care. If, as a society, we decide that we would prefer to spend 20 percent or more of our disposable income on medical care, is that wrong? University of Chicago professor of economics and Nobel Laureate Robert W. Fogel tries to place the debate about health care spending in the context of economic history.[32] He argues that, compared with the 19th century, human beings spend far fewer resources on basic necessities like food, clothing, and shelter. As a result, we have more resources for other things. He argues that the growth in spending on medical care is due to "the success of medical interventions combined with rising incomes."[33] In other words, we have more money to spend, and we are using it on technologies that have improved our lives, so perhaps this is not a problem.

The objection to this line of reasoning is that, despite what Fogel claims about the success of medical interventions, we are not spending these newly available resources well. In other words, are we generating "value for money"?[34] David Cutler, a health economist at Harvard University, argues that we should focus less on the level of health care expenditure and pay greater attention to whether or not the expenditures generate more benefits than costs.[35] Until the late 1960s, most people assumed that the "value question" was not an issue in the United States, but a growing body of research challenges this assumption.

One of the early pioneers in this area was Dr. Kerr White, a physician and economist who taught at the University of North Carolina and later at Johns Hopkins University. Dr. White helped to establish the field of health services research. He was the recipient of one of the first Hill-Burton Act grants for patient care research. As part of this study, he found that, in systems with better access to primary care, rates of hospitalizations were lower.[36] This work was taken up by White's student at Johns Hopkins University, Barbara Starfield, who went on to become one of the leaders in the field of health services research.[37]

White also influenced a young physician named John Wennberg and encouraged him to look at hospital discharge data.[38] In 1973, Wennberg, who was hired to be the director of Vermont's Regional Medical Program at the University of Vermont, and Alan Gittelsohn, Wennberg's former statistics professor at Johns Hopkins University, published a remarkable study of health care use and spending in Vermont. In their article, Wennberg and Gittelsohn documented wide, unexplained variations in medical resources, medical expenditures, and the use of medical care by thirteen different "hospital services areas" in Vermont. For example, they found that the rate of tonsillectomies in Vermont ranged from 13 in the lowest to 152 per 10,000 in the highest hospital service area. Although they were unable to measure differences in need or outcome directly, they argued that the magnitude of the differences they observed was unlikely to be explained by either. Physician uncertainty about the effectiveness of different treatments, rather than differences in rates of disease, explained the geographic variation they documented. They concluded that "there is considerable uncertainty about the aggregate, as well as specific kinds, of health care services."[39] In subsequent work, Wennberg and colleagues linked physician uncertainty to a lack of sufficient clinical evidence about alternative treatments. Researchers from the United States and around the world have continued to document such variation in subsequent decades.[40] The work documenting unexplained small-area variation in health care spending suggested that a lot of health spending did not represent good value—and this shifted the policy agenda considerably.

Similarly, research by Robert Brook and his colleagues at RAND in the late 1970s and early 1980s suggested that physicians were providing therapies to patients when scientific evidence did not support their use.[41] Commenting on the state of knowledge about variations in the use of medical care, Brook and colleagues claimed that "Even for services whose rates of use have been studied to some extent, we know relatively little about the association among indications for use, actual use, and eventual health outcomes"— and they challenged the medical profession and the government to invest in research that would provide better information about the appropriateness of medical care.[42] Findings from these studies raised new, troubling questions about whether medical care was being delivered on the basis of good evidence about an intervention's safety and effectiveness.

Expanding the Federal Government's Role in Health Technology Assessment

Concerns that many health care decisions were made with limited or contested evidence for doing so led various stakeholders—including physicians, researchers, health policy experts, and patient advocates—to promote the use of systematic and rigorous methods to obtain safety and effectiveness evidence about medical interventions, as well as to rate the quality of such evidence.[43] Policy makers responded to these concerns by increasing the capacity of the federal government to assess medical technologies. In particular, Kerr White pushed for the establishment of the National Center for Health Services Research (NCHSR) and was able to convince Phil Lee, the assistant secretary for health at the Department of Health, Education, and Welfare (HEW, now the Department of Health and Human Services), to support the idea. Lee's support, along with growing interest among policy makers in how federal money was being spent on the Medicare and Medicaid programs, led Congress to establish the NCHSR on May 2, 1968. The NCHSR's job was to focus on quality, access, costs, efficacy, and efficiency.

As Lee explained, "the ultimate goal of the Center is to aid practitioners and institutions involved in health services to improve the distribution and quality of services and to make the best possible use of manpower, funds and facilities. It seems to me that the mission of this Center is really the essence of what we are talking about when we refer to the formulation of public policy in the area of medical care."[44] Despite the initial excitement about the importance of the NCHSR's mission, it struggled to influence policy in what became an increasingly crowded field with several competing organizations and agencies. The NCHSR's budget remained stagnant at about $20 million, compared with about $6 billion for the National Institutes of Health (NIH), which funds basic science and human clinical trials that investigate the safety and effectiveness of medical drugs, biologics, and devices.[45]

In 1972, Congress established the Office of Technology Assessment (OTA) to advise federal lawmakers on science and technology policy, including the use of medical technologies. Between 1972 and 1995, the OTA produced reports for nearly every congressional committee, and through those reports, legislators could better understand new technologies and their policy implications. The reports helped set the terms of debate and increased understanding of the risks and implications of policy options.[46] Because these reports were designed to frame issues and assess multiple policy alternatives, they were often cited by both political parties during the same congressional debate.

In 1978, HEW created the National Center for Health Care Technology (NCHCT) to advise the Health Care Financing Administration (HCFA) on Medicare coverage issues. Only four years after its creation, the Reagan administration eliminated the NCHCT. The demise of this agency was driven in part by objections from industry and medical professionals. Opponents argued that the work of NCHCT represented inappropriate regulation of industry,[47] but it was also criticized by organized medicine because it threatened to challenge clinical judgment by introducing cost-effectiveness as a criterion for what interventions to offer patients.[48] Some of the work of the NCHCT was taken up by the NCHSR.

After eliminating the NCHCT, the Institute of Medicine (IOM) created the Council on Health Care Technology (CHCT) in 1986 in response to congressional concerns about the continued need for health technology assessment. The CHCT only conducted two formal evaluations, and the IOM did not seek additional funding for the program after 1989.[49] The Reagan administration's elimination of NCHCT, however, did not end congressional enthusiasm for health services research. Dr. John Wennberg, a professor of medicine at Dartmouth College and a pioneer in the study of small area variation in health care, had convinced several members of Congress that it was important to have better information about the quality of medical technologies. He argued that research on unexplained variations in the practice of medicine would allow the government to address the growth of Medicare and Medicaid spending by identifying unnecessary care.[50]

In an effort to increase the prominence of health services research and increase its funding, the NCHSR became the Agency for Health Care Policy and Research (AHCPR) in 1989. As Wennberg explained in a 1992 article, "the variations that exist between care of residents of New Haven and Boston, two of the nation's most medically sophisticated cities, were particularly useful in raising the 'which rate is right' question in the halls of Congress . . . I also made the point that the magnitude of the problem exposed by practice variations required a new initiative in federal science policy."[51] William Roper, who became administrator for the HCFA in 1986, promoted the use of Medicare databases to address some of these concerns by monitoring quality of care. Influenced by Wennberg, Roper, and others, several congressional leaders—including U.S. Senate Majority Leader George Mitchell (D-ME), Senator David Durenberger (R-MN), the ranking Republican on the Senate Finance Committee, and Representative Bill Gradison (R-OH), the ranking Republican on the Health Subcommittee of Ways and Means—heralded the idea that evidence-based approaches could save Medicare billions of dollars by identifying unnecessary health care services in high-cost areas without harming patients.[52] As Representative Gradison asserted, "Questions are being raised about the value of the outcomes of the expanding number of medical treatments."[53]

In response to these concerns, AHCPR was created in 1989 with bipartisan congressional and professional support to carry out outcomes studies, develop practice guidelines, and conduct and coordinate health services research. In the first few years of its operation, the agency established a new program for developing practice guidelines as well as 14 new Patient Outcomes Research Teams (PORTs), multidisciplinary centers focused on particular medical problems (e.g., back pain, myocardial infarction) to determine "what worked."[54] Inspired by the work of Wennberg and other researchers who had documented unexplained practice variation in the United States, the goal of the PORT program was to provide better evidence for clinical decision making and reduce variations in treatment practice. The agency gave priority to medical problems that were associated with expensive treatments and high levels of practice variation.

Political Attacks on Health Services Research

During the early 1990s, AHCPR frequently assisted the White House, under both the Bush and Clinton administrations, in assessing the implications of different health reform policy options. Although the leaders of the agency hoped that these efforts would demonstrate the value of AHCPR to policy makers, its association with the Clinton administration's health reform initiatives was later seen as a liability.

Despite some initial success, a broad government reduction agenda—the so-called "Contract with America"—was introduced in 1994 when the Republicans gained control of both the House and Senate, and the AHCPR's performance fell under significant scrutiny, to such an extent that it risked being eliminated during the 1996 budget appropriations. AHCPR's vulnerability to termination was attributable to many factors, several of which related to the strategies underlying its creation,[55] but the opposition of influential lobby groups also had a substantial effect. In particular, the North American Spine Society (NASS), an association of back surgeons, who, in collaboration with the Center for Patient Advocacy, mounted a serious attack on the agency in 1995 after its PORT on low-back pain concluded that "there was no evidence to support spinal-fusion surgery and that such surgery commonly had complications." A letter-writing campaign to gain congressional support was organized, and the NASS used personal contacts to obtain the backing of a number of Republican politicians.[56]

While the interest group attack made it difficult for the AHCPR to survive, the fact that the OTA was eliminated at the same time is evidence that the AHCPR was caught up in a broader attack on government-based policy research. Despite wide praise for the agency and its research, Congress eliminated the OTA's funding in 1995, following the 1994 midterm elections, in which the Republican party regained control of the House of Representatives. OTA, like AHCPR, was caught up in a broader effort to shrink the size of government, but it also came under criticism from some Republicans because, in some of its reports, the OTA questioned whether there was sufficient evidence to justify Medicare reimbursement for some medical technologies.[57] These findings alienated many stakeholders, including some within organized medicine and the drug and device industries.[58]

Unlike OTA, AHCPR benefitted from a series of behind-the-scenes negotiations that involved lobbying by the former members of Congress who helped to create the agency—along with the fact that many of the problems that underpinned its establishment remained (such as practice variations and cost concerns). Thanks to these negotiations, the agency survived, albeit with a new name, the Agency for Healthcare Research and Quality (AHRQ), that deliberately eliminated the word "policy," the abandonment of its practice guideline program, and a 21 percent budget cut.[59] As John Wennberg put it,

> the unfortunate political history of . . . AHCPR . . . illustrate[s] the risks
> inherent in efforts to evaluate the common practices . . . stable funding;
> strong peer review to assure good science and freedom from conflicts of
> interest that affect judgments; policies that sustain the careers of leading

scientists over a professional lifetime (keeping them free of dependency on funding from the drug and device companies whose products they evaluate); and deep commitment on the part of the scientific establishment sufficient to withstand the wrath of practitioners and others with vested interests who find their favorite theories slain by evidence or demand for their services reduced because informed patients want less.[60]

Even after the agency's near-death experience, many health policy experts—with support from some members of Congress—continued to push for studies to examine whether medical interventions were not only safe and therapeutically effective but cost-effective. These calls increased in the years immediately preceding the 2008 election.

Renewed Enthusiasm for Comparative Effectiveness Research

Political scientists who study agenda change often point to "focusing events" that alter the political landscape and lead directly to changes in the policy agenda.[61] Nothing had a more dramatic effect on the health policy agenda with regard to quality than two reports by the IOM. *To Err Is Human: Building a Safer Health Care System*, published in 1999, reported that preventable medical errors in U.S. hospitals resulted in an estimated 44,000 to 98,000 deaths each year.[62] *Crossing the Quality Chasm*, published two years later in 2001, generated a bit less media attention than *To Err is Human* but offered a comprehensive agenda for reform. The report called for improvements in health care safety, effectiveness, patient-centeredness, timeliness, efficiency, and equity. Its recommendations were consistent with many of the efforts by patient advocates because it tied quality issues "more closely to patients' experiences, cost, and social justice."[63] Together, these two reports fundamentally altered the policy debate and, as Vladeck and Rice put it, "leaders throughout the system are now paying appropriate attention" to the issues of safety and quality.[64]

The 2003 Medicare Modernization Act (MMA) authorized AHRQ to conduct and disseminate comparative effectiveness research to "improve the quality, effectiveness, and efficiency of health care" financed by public insurance programs.[65] For the AHRQ to accomplish this goal, the MMA established the Effective Health Care program to oversee a range of external research networks that conduct systematic evidence reviews to assess the effectiveness, comparative effectiveness, safety, and, in rare cases, cost-effectiveness of medical technologies and interventions.[66] Although establishing the program reflected congressional interest in comparative information on the value of health care interventions, the limitations placed on the new program also reflected the continued influence of industry on health technology assessment policy.[67] The legislation prohibited AHRQ from mandating national standards of clinical practice and banned CMS from using comparative effectiveness information produced by the Effective Health Care program to withhold or restrict access to prescription drugs.[68] Equally important, AHRQ's budget was reduced, and the agency received only $15 million to carry out its new responsibilities.

Advocacy for comparative effectiveness research emerged again during health reform efforts that led to passage of the ACA. In late 2006 and early 2007, a shift from a Republican to a Democratic congressional majority renewed the focus on health care and the need for comprehensive reform. Democratic members of Congress began to advocate for comparative effectiveness research as a mechanism to address quality by encouraging the use of evidence about medical technologies in clinical decision making. A 2007 House proposal called for a new comparative effectiveness research program within AHRQ. Senators Max Baucus (D-MT) and Kent Conrad (D-ND) introduced legislation (S. 3408) that would establish a nongovernmental, public-private entity, based on the idea that a nongovernmental body would offer a more efficient, transparent, and accepted mechanism to integrate comparative effectiveness research into U.S. health care decision making.[69] Neither proposal was adopted, but these ideas were incorporated into the ACA.

Interest in comparative effectiveness research continued to grow during the 2008 presidential campaign. Although comparative effectiveness research garnered bipartisan support in the campaign, once Obama was elected in November 2008 and the Democrats took control of both houses of Congress, Republican support waned, with many party leaders distancing themselves from or opposing the issue.[70] In fact, by the time the ACA was adopted in 2010, comparative effectiveness research was more partisan than ever. Many Republican members of Congress expressed fierce opposition to comparative effectiveness research, arguing that such research would lead to rationing of care and "cookbook medicine." They did not want findings of federally supported research about the effectiveness of medical technologies to lead to changes in clinical practice or payer coverage policies that would result in patients being denied access to medical technologies.

In the end, the ACA authorized the creation of a public-private research institute, PCORI, to identify research priorities, establish a research agenda, and fund comparative effectiveness research projects. However, to address fears that comparative effectiveness research would be used to ration health care, the ACA prohibits the use of quality-adjusted life years (QALYs) to reinforce the fact that consideration of costs would not be prescribed in the research and that findings published by PCORI would not dictate recommendations for payer coverage or health policy initiatives affecting patients' access to medical technologies and interventions.

To implement its mission, PCORI draws on a dedicated trust fund of dollars from the Medicare program and contributions from private insurers.

The ACA also provided substantial funding and remit to AHRQ to disseminate findings from comparative effectiveness research and to link databases and disease registries to improve the evidence base for the use of medical technologies. But at the same time, Congress limited the ability of CMS to use cost-effectiveness analysis in making decisions about what medical technologies Medicare will pay for,[71] and it inserted in the ACA limitations on CMS's use of findings from comparative effectiveness studies, in response to fears that the findings of these studies would be used to restrict patients' access to care, weaken physicians' autonomy, result in health care rationing, and threaten biomedical innovation.[72] One interpretation of the ACA restrictions is that they represent a continuation of a long history of congressional efforts to limit the Medicare program's ability to raise the evidentiary standards for medical technologies the program will pay for. As one commentator put it, "the creation of [PCORI] represents a challenging new chapter in America's on-again, off-again support for determining what works in health care."[73]

Soon after the creation of PCORI, Gail Wilensky, a health economist who has worked in several federal leadership positions, warned that "We're off to a good start, but the future of [comparative effectiveness research] is still fragile."[74] Recognizing PCORI's limited political support and hoping to avoid the problems that led to the demise of the OTA and attacks on AHCPR, the leadership at PCORI adopted a conservative approach to its work. A large percentage of PCORI's expenditures between 2011 and 2015 were for studies that addressed methodological questions related to evaluating medical technologies or for efforts to build stakeholder and broad public support for the organization's work. Although PCORI did fund several studies that compared the effectiveness of different treatments and some argued that its focus on patient concerns filled "a critical void,"[75] critics argued that PCORI was "timid" in its efforts to address inefficiencies in the health care system.[76]

By 2015, however, critics were becoming increasingly vocal about PCORI's lack of visible success. Topher Spiro of the Center for American Progress was quoted as saying that "if it doesn't prove its worth soon there will be increasing calls for getting rid of it, or reducing its funding."[77] Gail Wilensky argued that "PCORI seems to have become almost invisible. Maybe they think that's the best way to stay under the political radar screen," but it has not yet "offer[ed] much value."[78] As expected, Republicans in Congress were less generous with their assessments. That year, the House of Representatives attempted to abolish AHRQ and cut funding for PCORI in an attempt to rein in research that would provide more and better evidence about the effectiveness of medical technologies.[79] Unlike the House of Representatives, the U.S. Senate did not vote to abolish AHRQ, but in 2016 the Senate proposed a 35 percent cut to the agency's budget. However, with support from the Obama administration, this was reduced to 8 percent.[80]

The first proposed budget by President Trump also called for the elimination of AHRQ but provided $272 million to the NIH (about $60 million less than AHRQ's $334 million budget in the last year of the Obama administration), which might be used to support some of the research activities that AHRQ would have funded. The congressional restrictions on comparative effectiveness research and the lack of support by the Trump administration notwithstanding, public and private insurers are increasingly asking for evidence that medical technologies are effective in improving patient health outcomes before they agree to pay for those technologies.[81] Yet, as our cases illustrate, what constitutes adequate evidence of effectiveness remains deeply contested.[82] Furthermore, even when there is broad agreement that a medical technology is highly effective, as in the case of the newest generation of drugs to treat hepatitis C, there are important disputes about how to assess their value and set an appropriate price.

Medicare's Renewed Interest in Evidence of Effectiveness

Along with the expansion of the federal government's investment in comparative effectiveness research during the 1980s, there was growing concern about how the Medicare program was making coverage decisions. Amid growing complaints that its coverage process was unpredictable, unclear, and lengthy, in 1989 the HCFA (later CMS), under the Bush administration, pushed for regulations stating that for purposes of coverage, a technology would need to be safe, effective, noninvestigational, appropriate, and accepted by the medical community.[83] The inclusion of costs and cost-effectiveness as an explicit criterion in selected cases was also proposed, and this was the first time that HCFA had supported such considerations as criteria in coverage decisions. In the proposed regulations, HCFA argued that the existing Medicare law authorized the agency to consider cost when making coverage decisions. HCFA argued that the provisions in the legislation that created the Medicare program stating that covered costs should be "reasonable" encompassed the authority for the program "to consider cost as a factor in making Medicare coverage decisions."[84] The proposed regulation generated substantial opposition from medical and industry groups, including the AMA and the Pharmaceutical Research and Manufacturers Association of America, who feared that important technologies would be rationed, leaving seniors to pay for or forgo necessary care, and was eventually withdrawn.[85] HFCA tried to revive the effort to include cost-effectiveness again in the mid-1990s, but it was again opposed by representatives of industry and Republican leaders in Congress. In light of this opposition, HCFA director Bruce Vladeck decided not to pursue cost-effectiveness and told Congress that "manufacturers or providers do not need to submit formal cost-effectiveness analyses to HCFA in order to have a service considered for coverage."[86]

In 2000, at the end of the Clinton administration, the HCFA issued a notice of intent (NOI) to publish a proposal that would introduce the concept of "added value" into coverage decisions.[87] The proposed standards would require that new technologies provide some benefits to beneficiaries beyond what was already available to them in the program. If a technology did not provide added value, Medicare would deny coverage. The costs of alternative treatment options were therefore clearly being considered relevant to determining coverage. As with the previous attempts to introduce cost-effectiveness into coverage decisions, negative comments on the NOI persuaded the Department of Health and Human Services (HHS) and HCFA to withdraw this proposal, and no further attempt was made to address these issues through regulation.[88]

Beyond the issue of cost-effectiveness, CMS has been limited in its capacity to use evidence for making coverage decisions because there are significant gaps in the available evidence bases, particularly as related to older and disabled Medicare beneficiaries, who are usually not included in clinical trials. In part to address this issue, in 2006 CMS issued guidance on a new policy called "coverage with evidence development" (CED). The aim is to give some beneficiaries access to potentially promising technologies where available evidence on their clinical effectiveness is either insufficient or restricted to a particular patient population. The evidence is to be obtained from the use of the technology with relevant Medicare patients enrolled in prospective clinical studies or data about clinical use with Medicare patients submitted to an approved registry.[89] Unlike previous attempts to codify the role of evidence in the CMS's coverage policies, CED has largely escaped political backlash through its framing as a mechanism to enhance the adoption of new therapies, rather than to control or slow their diffusion,[90] and because it avoided the issue of cost-effectiveness. Moreover, the policy has been applied in a limited number of cases since its inception, thereby lessening any perceived threat. For example, despite available comparative effectiveness evidence demonstrating that computed tomography of the coronary arteries offers little advantage over current angiographic approaches, the CMS has not been able to stop paying for the procedure, due to strong resistance by radiologists.[91]

In addition to the fact that CMS has only applied the CED process to a small number of technologies, the data it has required to make such determinations has varied considerably over the years.[92] Given the problems with the program, in 2011 the agency announced a plan to rewrite the policy, and by November 2012 it issued draft guidance on CED. The 2012 guidance limited the scope of CED to "coverage with study participation," which involves gathering of data when an intervention was deemed reasonable and necessary only for patients enrolled in clinical studies designed to provide reliable evidence of its health benefits and risks.[93]

The case of PET scans for detecting amyloid beta plaque in the living brain is one recent example of the use of CED to say no to routine coverage of a new technology, but it is not clear how frequently CMS will invoke CED or how many resources will be dedicated to these efforts. Not surprisingly, the policy has faced some opposition from patient advocacy groups as well as from manufacturers, who argue that CED raises the threshold of evidence needed to obtain a positive coverage determination and slows access to medical advances.[94]

Evidence of Value for Private Payers

The efforts by HCFA and CMS to become value-based purchasers were, in many respects, preceded by the private sector. Because the United States relies, for many people under the age of 65, on an employer-based health insurance system, corporate leaders began pursuing mechanisms for improving the quality of medical care they were purchasing for their employees. By the mid-1980s, many large employers had turned to managed care to help control health care costs. Under this approach, insurers contract with a managing company to monitor the cost of treatments, and patients are restricted to specific physicians and hospitals from which they receive medical care. Several Fortune 500 companies, including Bank of America, Ford, General Motors, and Xerox, wanted better information about the quality of medical care they were paying for through their company health plans. In response, the National Committee for Quality Assurance (NCQA), worked with corporate leaders to develop standards for health plans employers offered to their employees.

NCQA was established in 1979 at the request of the federal Office for Health Maintenance Organizations and by the Group Health Association of America and the American Association of Foundations for Medical Care. In 1988, NCQA reorganized itself and created a board that included representatives of corporations, consumers, and quality experts. Health plans are still on the NCQA board, but they are a minority. NCQA developed accreditation standards for health plans in 1991. In 1993, NCQA started publishing report cards based on the Healthcare Effectiveness Data and Information Set. Today, NCQA publishes health plan report cards in *Consumer Reports*.

In theory, health plan report cards allow corporations, public purchasers, and individuals to compare plans on the basis of comparable quality measures. There is little evidence, however, that people "vote with their feet" and select health plans on the basis of health plan report cards.[95] Elbel and Schlesinger found that even when patients experience significant problems with their plans, most people "do not formally voice their complaints or exit health plans."[96] These findings are consistent with a number of studies that evaluate the use of safety and quality information by the public. In 1988, for example, Bruce Vladeck found that the publication of hospital mortality data did not influence the selection of hospitals by patients or physicians who refer them.[97] More recent assessments of the response to quality information have reached similar conclusions.[98]

Along with corporate efforts to measure and disseminate information about health care and health plan quality, private health insurance companies themselves have adopted policies designed to promote greater value. As with public payers, private health insurance companies are continually trying to manage "conflicts between the desire to speed the adoption of new medical technologies and the need to keep health insurance affordable."[99] The concept of medical necessity is key to these conflicts. Private health insurance companies do not have to cover technologies or services if there isn't sufficient evidence that these interventions will generate a clinical benefit and, since the 1970s, private insurance companies have been requiring physicians and hospitals to justify their services in terms of medical necessity.[100] But the term medical necessity is rarely defined and is frequently a source of disagreement.[101] For example, in recent years, many patients who have been prescribed a direct-acting antiviral agent to treat chronic hepatitis C virus have been denied coverage by an insurer. Although these denials are more common among patients on Medicaid, patients with private health insurance have experienced a denial as well. The most common reasons for denial of treatment "were insufficient information to assess medical need (134 [35.5 percent]) and lack of medical necessity (132 [35.0 percent])."[102]

Conclusion

Everyone wants the preventive, diagnostic, or treatment interventions they use to work for the intended purpose—and to be affordable. Yet many policy initiatives to ensure that medical technologies work, that some are better than others, and that they are cost-effective have been attacked, scaled back, and eliminated in response to claims the policies would stifle innovation and limit which technologies physicians can offer their patients. Looming over the debates about getting better evidence regarding the value of medical technologies is the rhetorical and political power that comes from implicit and explicit claims that initiatives to improve the quality and value of medical technologies will lead to health care rationing. And as the remaining chapters illustrate, questions about how to get better evidence about quality and value, about who should be involved in evidence gathering, and about what kind of evidence to obtain and how to evaluate it are linked to political, ideological, and economic factors that do not always align with party identification or professional identities. They are also questions that will continue to generate intense debate in the wake of current transformations in the United States regarding health care delivery, patients' access to health insurance, and the cost of medical technologies.

CHAPTER THREE

Mammography Screening: Vested Interests and Polarization

Mammography screening is broadly regarded as an important tool in the fight against breast cancer, but the emphasis on mammography screening for reducing breast cancer mortality and the value of mammography screening among younger women have been debated for decades. In 2009, in the midst of the U.S. debate over the ACA, the USPSTF issued new guidelines that recommended against routine mammography screening for women ages 40 to 49 and called for biennial, rather than annual, screening among older women. The recommendations suggested that younger women should have the option to be screened after considering the benefits and harms with their physician. This was not the first time scientists had questioned the value of mammography screening, particularly for younger women, nor was it the first time such debates had generated controversy. Nevertheless, the USPSTF's recommendations became fodder for a highly contentious fight about the meaning of health reform, the appropriate role of the government (or even private organizations providing recommendations to government departments, like USPSTF) with regard to clinical recommendations and, more broadly, how to evaluate the benefits and harms of medical technology.

The controversy over mammography screening is part of the larger debate we address in this book. How can we make sense of evidence, and how should it be used to make decisions about the use of medical care technology? Understanding the mammography screening debate offers a useful window into the politics of medical care technology in the United States. It illustrates the way disagreements about evidence, fights among powerful interest groups and ideological divisions about the appropriate role of government, and the extent to which individual patients and physicians should control decisions about health care all intersect to shape decisions about medical technologies.

On one level, the debate about mammography screening reflects disagreements about evidence. How much should we weight evidence from controlled clinical trials compared with observational studies? What counts as a benefit, and what counts as a burden? When evaluating the benefits and burdens of an intervention like mammography screening, how should we compare the potential psychological burden of a false-positive diagnosis against a reduction in mortality? This case study, however, highlights the degree to which the answers to these questions are inextricably linked to economic and political interests. There is a large, wealthy, and influential coalition of interest groups that benefit from the continued use of mammography screening as a primary tool in the fight against breast cancer (many of whom have a stake in promoting screening, more generally, as a tool for combatting cancer and other diseases). In addition, the success of the campaign to link mammography screening to the fight against breast cancer makes it difficult to challenge the technology. Elected officials often treat support for mammography as evidence of their support for women and women's health. In the case of the 2009 recommendations, the effort to reduce the use of mammography screening among younger women took place in the middle of a major debate about health reform in which opponents were searching for evidence that expanded government involvement in the health care system would lead to unwarranted "rationing" and "death panels."[1] This led, inaccurately but predictably, to claims that the mammography screening recommendations were part of a larger effort by the government to interfere with the practice of medicine and reduce the choices available to patients.

Breast Cancer Trends in the United States

Skin and breast cancer are the two most common types of cancer in American women. In 2017, more than 250,000 women (and nearly 2,500 men) will receive a new diagnoses of invasive breast cancer in the United States.[2] Based on data from 2012 to 2014, 12.4 percent of women in the United States will be diagnosed with breast cancer in their lifetime.[3] As of January 1, 2016, there were more than 3.5 million women in the United States with a history of breast cancer, including women who are cancer-free and others who are living with the disease.[4]

The incidence of breast cancer rose dramatically in the 1980s and 1990s. Some of the increase was due to heightened longevity and higher levels of obesity, but the findings were due primarily to increases in the use of mammography screening rather than an underlying change in the prevalence of the disease in the population. The prevalence of breast cancer and deaths associated with the disease have been declining since 2000.[5] These declines are often attributed to a combination of changes in lifestyle, earlier detection, and advances in treatment. In response to claims that declines in prevalence and death can be attributed to the increasing use of mammography screening during the 1980s and 1990s, many suggest that other factors may be responsible, since the declines started before population statistics would have revealed mammography's effect.[6]

As with many health and health care outcomes in the United States, aggregate improvements mask stark inequalities.[7] Decades of research has documented large socioeconomic inequalities in cancer mortality within the United States. In particular, black women have significantly higher rates of mortality due to breast cancer than other racial or ethnic groups.[8] In fact, one study of breast cancer mortality among the 50 largest cities in the United States found growing black-white disparities in breast cancer mortality between 1990 and 2009 because mortality rates have fallen much faster among whites.[9] Mortality rates are also higher among people who live in more deprived neighborhoods.[10] The large and growing demographic differences such as race and socioeconomic level in breast cancer mortality are not well understood, but they appear to be due to a wide range of factors, including inequalities in health behaviors and health care. In 2012, the National Cancer Institute (NCI) launched a new study "to find the underlying causes of breast cancer in black women, and to better understand why they are more likely to die of breast cancer than are white women."[11] The NCI project includes a $12 million grant to understand the degree to which genetics contribute to high rates of breast cancer deaths among black women.

Breast Cancer Advocacy and the Role of Mammography Screening

Before the 1970s, breast cancer was rarely discussed in public and largely ignored by the media, policymakers, and the general public. A number of prominent women began to change the public's awareness and perception of the disease. In 1971, Marvella Bayh, the wife of Senator Birch Bayh (R-IN), announced that she had breast cancer. She was followed in 1972 by actress and politician Shirley Temple Black.[12] The 1973 book *Our Bodies, Ourselves*,[13] published by the Boston Women's Health Book Collective, also raised awareness, but the willingness of First Lady Betty Ford and Governor Nelson A. Rockefeller's wife, Happy, to announce that they had undergone mastectomies inspired other women to share their experiences.[14] In 1974, First Lady Betty Ford's announcement that she had undergone a mastectomy is associated with an increase in breast cancer detection rates known as the "Betty Ford blip."[15]

Along with increasing public awareness, newspaper coverage, and medical journal articles on breast cancer, public announcements by prominent women of their breast cancer diagnosis set in motion several campaigns to raise money for research and advocacy. For example, Rose Kushner, journalist and preeminent breast cancer activist, led a successful campaign in the mid-1970s to end one-step Halsted radical mastectomy and in the 1980s turned her attention to the use of chemotherapy for postmenopausal women with breast cancer. In 1984, she wrote an article criticizing this practice and advocated for the use of tamoxifen, an antiestrogen compound that had fewer side effects. Many oncologists disagreed with her interpretation of the data and thought her writings would discourage women who could benefit from adjuvant chemotherapy from seeking this treatment. Although tamoxifen was later recognized by the FDA as standard therapy for postmenopausal women with positive lymph nodes and estrogen-receptor-positive breast cancers, Kushner's relationship with the drug's manufacturer raises important ethical questions that continue to be relevant today. Although no one raised concerns about conflicts of interest at the time, Kushner and her breast cancer advisory committee accepted substantial donations from Stuart Pharmaceuticals.[16] Today, this sort of potential conflict of interest would be viewed as troubling. Indeed, critics are concerned that the pharmaceutical industry continues to have too much influence on breast cancer advocates.

The Susan G. Komen Foundation (known today as Susan G. Komen) was founded in 1982, and the National Alliance of Breast Cancer Organizations, a large umbrella organization with hundreds of members, was established in 1986.[17] During the 1990s, the National Breast Cancer Coalition, Breast Cancer Action, and several local breast cancer support organizations were established. In addition to providing support to women with breast cancer, these organizations encouraged political activism to find a cure and improve treatment. These efforts resulted in a quadrupling of federal dollars for breast cancer research during the decade. The National Breast Cancer Coalition convinced Congress to channel "more than one billion dollars for breast cancer research through the Department of Defense"[18]

If anything, the success of breast cancer advocates in raising money for their cause has generated concern among public health officials and advocates for other diseases. Indeed, the case of patient advocacy for breast cancer research and treatment remind us that "successful" advocacy on the part of patient organizations, particularly when they focus on a specific disease, is not necessarily desirable public policy. Heart disease and lung cancer both contribute to more deaths among woman than breast cancer, but neither research funding nor public awareness reflect this. Funding for research, treatment, and education should not necessarily reflect, in a linear fashion, the number of people affected by a disease or its contribution to the mortality rate, but as Brower argues, "How the issue—and fear—of breast cancer came to occupy such a prominent place in the consciousness of women worldwide, while lung cancer stealthily became the new killer, illustrates the power of public relations campaigns and patient activism."[19]

The advocacy groups that started in the 1980s grew steadily in the 1990s and mobilized a large network of patients, families, and friends to generate public awareness and raise money.[20] Susan G. Komen in particular led the way to work with industry on cause marketing partnerships. Corporate sponsors offer support for Komen's public awareness campaigns and research efforts and, in return, they improve their public image by supporting what is perceived to be a public good.[21] For example, since 1991, the athletic footwear and apparel company New Balance has sponsored Komen's Race for the Cure, and the company donates 5 percent of the retail price of athletic shoes to Komen.[22] These efforts generated significant support for breast cancer research and treatment.[23] Approximately $6 billion per year is spent on breast cancer research awareness campaigns.[24] In contrast to many other diseases, including other forms of cancer, funding for breast cancer is much higher when examined as a ratio of funding to disease incidence, mortality, or potential years of life lost, leading critics to argue that breast cancer is now "over funded."[25]

Advocacy has also helped fuel remarkable improvements in the treatment of the disease. Evolution in the technology of breast cancer treatment has been significant. While the vast majority of breast cancer patients receive some sort of surgery, the nature of the surgery has changed dramatically. In the 1950s and '60s, surgeons assumed that removing more tissue was the key to reducing the risk of reoccurrence and mortality.[26] Whereas previously, surgical intervention meant complete removal of the breast through mastectomy, breast-conserving surgery, such as lumpectomy, is now used more frequently. Following clinical indications, such surgery is often combined with radiotherapy, chemotherapy, and/or hormone therapy to prevent relapse in the remaining breast tissue.

Advances have occurred in chemotherapy, particularly with regard to breast cancer treatment.[27] New drugs have been developed to stop cancer cell growth, and improvements have been made in the way existing drugs are administered, including adjustments in frequency of dosage, drug combinations, and an increase focus on neoadjuvant therapy, or prior to surgery, in order to reduce the size of the tumor, facilitating breast conservation.[28] Chemotherapy may also be used in adjuvant treatment, along with or instead of radiation therapy, to prevent relapse. In more recent years, a variety of new antibody drugs have been used to target breast cancers with a growth-promoting protein known as HER2/neu on their surface. The use of these targeted HER2 antibody therapies can improve survival in some breast cancer patients, although some cancers develop resistance to these treatments and require additional and coadjuvant therapies.[29]

Although some forms of breast cancer respond well to chemotherapy of new targeted drugs, about two-thirds of breast cancers are hormone receptor–positive (ER-positive or PR-positive) and respond effectively to hormone therapy. Hormone therapy was first introduced in the late 1970s. For example, tamoxifen, which blocks the actions of estrogen, is now widely used instead of or in addition to chemotherapy, especially among older women. The development of a new type of hormone therapy, aromatase inhibitors, which block the production of estrogen, is another advancement in the way that breast cancer is treated.

Mammography Screening

The origin of mammography screening is more than a century old. In 1913, a German surgeon named Albert Salomon at the University of Berlin used radiography to identify the spread of tumors to ancillary lymph nodes in mastectomy specimens.[30] There was little additional attention to the potential for using radiography to detect breast cancer until 1930, when Dr. Stafford Warren from Rochester Memorial Hospital in Rochester, New York, used new film from Kodak and Patterson, intensifying screens to perform mammography on 119 women who later underwent surgery for breast cancer. In all but eight cases, the mammography was able to help accurately diagnose the patient. For the next several decades, clinicians in Europe and the United States continued to develop and use improved mammography techniques and equipment for the purpose of improving the clarity of images and reducing exposure to radiation.[31] By the early 1960s, clinicians also began to advocate for the routine use of mammography screening in asymptomatic women,[32] and the NCI funded a trial to investigate the use of mammography to screen for breast cancer [33]

Today, the overwhelming consensus among leading breast cancer advocacy groups—and within the clinical literature—is that mammography screening reduces breast cancer mortality. A review of the literature on mammography screening published in 2014 in the *Journal of the American Medical Association* (*JAMA*) concluded that "Mammography screening is associated with a 19% overall reduction of breast cancer mortality (approximately 15% for women in their 40s and 32% for women in their 60s)."[34] But the same article also noted that "For a 40- or 50-year-old woman undergoing 10 years of annual mammograms, the cumulative risk of a false-positive result is about 61%."[35] Similarly, a 2015 article published in *JAMA* based on a systematic review of the literature found that "across all ages at average risk, screening was associated with a reduction in breast cancer mortality of approximately 20%," but there was uncertainty about the magnitude of benefit associated with annual and biennial screening among women age 40 to 49.[36]

The evidence from controlled clinical trials regarding the benefits of mammography screening is more ambiguous. The first clinical trial to examine the benefits of mammography screening was the 1963 New York Health Insurance Plan study. The trial involved 60,000 women aged 40 to 64 who were randomized, without informed consent, into two groups of 30,000 each. The intervention group received annual two-view mammography screens and clinical breast exams. The control group received "usual" care.[37] The trial found that mammography was associated with a 23 percent reduction in breast cancer mortality compared with the control group but found no benefit among women age 40 to 49.

During the 1970s and 1980s, several more clinical trials, using different methodological approaches, produced mixed results regarding the impact of mammography screening on mortality. Multiple trials in Canada and the United Kingdom using randomization at the individual level found no statistically significant impact of mammography on breast cancer mortality.[38] A two-county study in Sweden that began in 1977 involved 76,000 women age 40 to 74 (39,000 in the intervention group and 37,500 in the control group), which used geographic-cluster randomization, rather than individual randomization, into the intervention and control groups, found that single-view mammography was associated with a statistically significant 32 percent reduction in breast cancer mortality at the 12-year follow-up—but the 14-year follow-up found no differences for women age 40 to 49.[39]

Proponents of mammography argue that, along with data from clinical trials, there is a substantial amount of evidence from observational studies that demonstrate the value of screening.[40] Despite the strong support for mammography, a number of experts argue that it has been oversold. Most breast cancer survivors received a mammogram and attribute their survival to the screen, but critics contend that most of these cancers could have been cured anyway, even if they had been detected late.[41] In addition, many studies have failed to account fully for the negative effects of false positives.[42] They argue that public health campaigns have exaggerated the benefits of mammography screening and downplayed the benefits. Furthermore, they have relied on emotional appeals and the flawed logic that a test that offers a benefit to women age 50 and over must also be valuable to younger women.[43]

Concerns About Underuse and Overuse of Screening

There is a continual push by public health organizations, professional associations, patient advocacy groups, academics, and clinicians to increase the use of screening—and a concern that its use is currently inadequate.[44] In the 1970s, the American Cancer Society's public health message was that "if you have not had a mammography, you need more than your breast examined."[45] More than 40 years later, the basic message has not changed. Susan G. Komen has funded ads urging women to "get screened now" because "early detection saves lives."[46] One hypothesis to explain the persistent black-white differences in breast cancer mortality, for example, is that black women are less likely to receive mammography screening or less likely to receive "adequately sequential" mammograms.[47] A study published in 2017, which compared women age 40 to 74 who had breast cancer that was detected by mammography screening with women with nonscreen-detected breast cancers found that rates of mastectomy and chemotherapy were 20 percent lower among women who had been detected by mammography. The authors concluded that "screening mammography decreases the extent of local and systemic treatment for breast cancer."[48]

Even among strong proponents of mammography, there is a recognition that it is an imperfect technology. Mammography is unable to identify certain types of breast cancer, including estrogen-receptor-negative cancers. In addition, there are large numbers of false positives, particularly among younger women. Mammography often identifies noninvasive cancers that would not require subsequent intervention if left undetected.[49] As Jatoi and Miller[50] explain, many impalpable cancers are indolent and unlikely to be malignant. Improvements in mammography technology make it more likely to detect breast tissue anomalies. One study estimated that, over the 30-year period between 1978 and 2008, more than a million women were overdiagnosed with breast cancer due to mammography.[51]

The debate over the potential harms of mammography, particularly among younger women, began relatively soon after its use became widespread in the United States in the late 1970s. Growing concerns about whether mammography was being overused led the NCI in 1993 to review available data on the consequences of mammography screening. It concluded that mammography helped to reduce deaths among women age 50 and over, but the evidence of benefit for women age 40 to 49 was unclear, and it recommended that women speak with their doctors about whether to undergo screening. NCI director Dr. Richard Klausner asserted that, for women in their forties, "the data are complex and the evidence is not transparent." The Clinton administration embraced the NCI's recommendations, though the president tried to anticipate the possibility that some insurance companies would use the recommendations as a reason not to cover mammography screening among younger women. President Clinton said that the federal government was doing "its part to make sure women have both coverage and access to this potentially life-saving test" and challenged "private health insurance plans to do the same. They, too, should cover regular screening mammograms for women 40 and over."[52]

Several physician organizations, including the American College of Physicians and the American Academy of Family Physicians, and most European countries, agreed with the position of the NCI. Other organizations, including the AMA, the National Cancer Society, and the American College of Radiology, disagreed with this position and continued to recommend routine mammography screening for younger women.[53] In 1996, in response to the scientific disagreement over the NCI recommendation, coupled with a new clinical trial conducted in Sweden that provided some evidence that mammography screening may be associated with statistically significant reduction in breast cancer deaths, Dr. Klausner called for a consensus conference to discuss the evidence.

In 1997, the NIH held the Consensus Development Conference on Breast Cancer Screening for Women Age 40–49. The conference brought together a large number of stakeholders, including representatives of the major clinical organizations in the United States. After two days of deliberation, the NIH conference issued a consensus statement that was similar to the 1993 NCI recommendations. The statement indicated that "informed decision making," rather than a recommendation of regular mammography screening among younger women, was appropriate.[54] Many radiologists criticized the panel for its statement and argued that this process was biased.[55]

There was extensive media coverage of the recommendations, and on February 4, 1997, the U.S. Senate adopted a nonbinding resolution, by a vote of 98–0, calling on the National Cancer Advisory Board (NCAB), an advisory board made up of 18 experts appointed by the president that provides advice to the director of the NCI about its programs and policies, to endorse routine mammography screening for women age 40 to 49.[56] The next day, the Subcommittee on Departments of Labor, Health and Human Services, and Education, and Related Agencies of the U.S. Senate Committee on Appropriations held a hearing to discuss the issue.[57] In a lengthy opening statement, Senator Arlen Spector (R-PA) argued that the NIH consensus conference had placed the burden of proof on those who promote the use of mammography screening among younger women.

When I took a look at the conclusions as they were reported, there was not enough evidence to conclude that women in their forties would benefit from mammograms as a part of routine health screening, the converse question occurred to me, which is this: is there sufficient evidence to conclude that women in their forties would not benefit from mammograms as a part of their routine health screening. If you put the burden of proof on saying that the medical evidence has to establish a benefit, as opposed to the evidence being inconclusive or in equipoise, with a very substantial body of evidence saying that the mammograms are very important, then it seems to me that we are allowing the burden of proof issue to dominate, with so much evidence, although perhaps inconclusive or perhaps even in equipoise as to whether it is a matter of benefit.[58]

On February 26, the Appropriations Subcommittee of the House Labor, Health and Human Services, and Education Committee also held a hearing on the mammography screening issue. Representative Porter (R-IL) questioned Dr. Klausner about the implications of the NIH recommendation for poor women under the age of 50. In the subsequent months, several members of Congress wrote letters to pressure Dr. Klausner and NCI to clarify its position on mammography screening.

One month later, in March 1997, the American Cancer Society held a workshop designed to discuss the controversy over screening guidelines. The majority of those invited to attend the workshop had already expressed preferences for universal screening, and the recommendations following the workshop reflected this conclusion. Based in part on the recommendation from the American Cancer Society workshop—coupled with pressure from Congress, the White House, and some advocacy groups—the NCAB issued a recommendation that the NCI should advise women age 40 to 49 at average risk for breast cancer to undergo mammography screening every year or two.[59] Soon after, the American Cancer Society and the NCI issued "A Joint Statement on Breast Cancer Screening for Women in Their 40s." The statement mentioned the limitations of screening but called for universal screening of women in their forties. The Clinton White House quickly moved to endorse the recommendation, and HHS Secretary Donna Shalala held a briefing at which she claimed, "Today, years of confusion have been replaced by clear, consistent scientific recommendation for women between the ages of 40 to 49."[60]

Despite the suggestion of scientific consensus, the bipartisan effort to encourage mammography screening in younger women who are not at elevated risk for breast cancer ignored growing disagreement among experts that this was an appropriate recommendation. It did reflect the political power of groups with a stake in mammography screening and the desire of both major political parties to highlight their concern for women's health. Republicans in Congress, only three years removed from helping to defeat President Clinton's proposal for national health insurance, viewed support for mammography screening as an opportunity to promote their support for women's health. Similarly, Democrats were eager to counter charges that they supported "rationing" of needed care and government interference with clinical decision making.

The 1997 NCI recommendation did not end the debate about early screening. Just five years later, in 2002, the USPSTF, an independent volunteer panel of 16 national experts in prevention and evidence-based medicine, continued to recommend routine mammography screening among women age 40 to 49, but the task force included language that urged clinicians to tell women that the benefits of mammography were smaller at younger ages.

The 2009 Mammography Screening Recommendations

Section 2713 of the ACA reads, "[F]or the purposes of this Act, and for the purposes of any other provision of law, the current recommendations of the United States Preventive Service Task Force (USPSTF) regarding breast cancer screening, mammography, and prevention shall be considered the most current other than those issued in or around November 2009."[61] This section of the ACA instructs agencies that are responsible for promulgating regulations under the law to accept recommendations of the USPSTF but to ignore one of its specific evidence-based practice recommendations regarding the use of mammography screening among women between the ages of 40 and 49.

The peculiar legislative language included in the ACA was a response by Congress to a 2009 recommendation of the USPSTF on the use of screening mammograms among younger women. In November 2009, the USPSTF published new recommendations about routine breast cancer screening mammography.[62] If followed, the new recommendations would reduce substantially the use of the procedure among women 40 to 49 years old.[63]

The 2009 recommendations, which replaced the guidance issued in 2002, were based on a detailed review and analysis of the relevant research. They called for the continuation of routine screening mammography among women age 50 and over but not for younger women who had no specific risk factors. The USPSTF explained that "for biennial screening mammography in women aged 40 to 49 years, there is moderate certainty that the net benefit is small"[64] and that the harms associated with breast cancer screening outweighed the benefits. These harms include "psychological harms, unnecessary imaging tests, biopsies in women without cancer, and inconvenience due to false-positive screening results." They also include "harms associated with treatment of cancer that would not have become clinically apparent during a woman's lifetime (overdiagnosis), as well as the harms of unnecessary earlier treatment of breast cancer that would have become clinically apparent but would not have shortened a woman's life."[65] The recommendations emphasized that the decision about mammography screening among younger women should depend on individual risk factors and a discussion between patients and their physicians about how to weight benefits and harms. As the chair of USPSTF, Dr. Albert Sui, argued after the task force reaffirmed its 2009 recommendations in 2015, "Women who place a higher value on the potential benefit than the potential harms [of screening mammography] may choose to begin biennial screening between the ages of 40 and 49 years."[66] He went on to explain that the grade of C was not a recommendation against screening, but "reflects moderate certainty of a net benefit or screening that is small in magnitude."[67]

The USPSTF enjoys a reputation for independence and quality.[68] It was established by HHS in 1984 during the Reagan administration, and since 1988 has operated under the authority of AHRQ (and its predecessor, the Agency for Health Care Policy and Research). Charged with developing recommendations on clinical preventive services, the USPSTF conducts a systematic review of all evidence about a preventive technology, assesses its benefits and harms, determines the certainty and magnitude of net benefit, and assigns a letter grade of A, B, C, or D to the preventive service under review. It is an independent volunteer panel of national experts in primary care, prevention, and evidence-based medicine, including people with backgrounds in internal medicine, family medicine, pediatrics, behavioral health, obstetrics and gynecology, and nursing.

Some responses to the USPSTF's 2009 mammography recommendations were positive. Groups such as Breast Cancer Action, the National Women's Health Network, the National Breast Cancer Coalition, and Our Bodies Ourselves embraced the recommendations. The recommendations were touted by some leading health policy researchers as "rational"[69] and "objective."[70] In response to claims that the USPSTF had made health care spending a "core concern" when writing the guidelines, Princeton economist Uwe Reinhardt asserted that the task force had conducted "a straightforward clinical-effectiveness analysis" that involved exploring "the pros and cons of a particular clinical approach strictly in terms of its positive and negative clinical consequences, not in terms of dollar outlays."[71] Wilensky also argued that the recommendations were based on a careful review of the evidence but accused the task force members as being "completely politically tone-deaf" for not anticipating the reaction to the new recommendations.[72] Indeed, the positive responses to the recommendations were overwhelmed by an avalanche of negative reactions from professional associations, patient advocates, and elected officials from both political parties.[73] Some of the opposition came from organizations with obvious economic interests, including radiologists, who were nearly unanimous in their condemnation of the recommendations. As one observer noted, if all women age 40 to 49 received an annual mammography screen, it would provide millions of dollars in revenue to radiologists and others, particularly when taking into consideration additional revenue generated by women with abnormal tests who require additional diagnostic work.[74]

Along with negative reaction from radiologists, strong objections came from some advocacy organizations like the American Cancer Society, which continued to recommend annual screening among women 45 years and over. Komen responded by claiming that "there is enough uncertainty about the age at which mammography should begin and the frequency of screening that we would not want to see a change in policy for screening mammography at this time."[75] Objections also came from within the medical profession.

Former NIH director Bernadine Healy, MD, said on Fox News, "I'm saying very powerfully [to] ignore [the recommendations], because unequivocally . . . this will increase the number of women dying of breast cancer."[76]

Some political leaders also responded with strong criticism. Within two weeks of their release, HHS Secretary Sebelius decried the "confusion and worry" the recommendations had stimulated and noted that the USPSTF does not "set federal policy and [doesn't] determine what services are covered by the federal government." She advised women to "Keep doing what you have been doing for years—talk to your doctor about your individual history, ask questions, and make the decision that is right for you."[77] Within a month, the Senate agreed by voice vote to an amendment that effectively required the federal government to ignore the task force's recommendations.[78] A slightly altered form of the amendment was included in the final version of the ACA.

The Problem with Disinvestment

It is not unprecedented for new practice guidelines to generate powerful opposition, as when the very funding of the AHCPR was successfully attacked in 1996, in part because of political objections to practice guidelines regarding back surgery.[79] Similarly, recommendations from the Medicare Payment Advisory Commission, particularly those that call for payment reductions, are also criticized regularly by stakeholders.[80] Even so, an important point about such controversies regarding practice guidelines is that they have been unusual. Several hundred new or revised practice guidelines are added every year to AHRQ's National Guideline Clearinghouse, which now catalogues about 2,400 guidelines, few of which have attracted any public concern.

So why the controversy over the USPSTF mammography screening recommendations? Findings from comparative-effectiveness research and other studies examining a technology's safety and effectiveness are often challenged when they result in calls for some degree of "disinvestment," that is, reducing the use of an established technology.[81] In fact, it may be more difficult to reduce or even eliminate the existing technologies than to block new technologies from reaching the market in the first place. This is consistent with research in political science on the mobilization of interest groups when existing policies and programs are threatened. Once a policy is adopted or a new program is created,[82] that policy automatically creates a constituency that benefits from its existence.[83] Because spending on existing technologies represents a source of income for many people, efforts to eliminate that technology will almost always generate some opposition. In the case of mammography screening, not only do the manufacturers of the equipment and the radiologists and other professionals who use it benefit from the continued and expanded use of this technology, so do a number of patient and other public health advocacy organizations. Work in behavioral economics also supports the idea that efforts at disinvestment in existing technologies would be particularly difficult. Behavioral economists have demonstrated that people respond more powerfully to a loss than they do to a gain.[84] This idea, known as "loss aversion," suggests that health care interest groups may view efforts by policymakers to take away existing benefits (or eliminate existing technologies) a less tolerable change than a failure to achieve initial approval for a technology that would deliver the same amount of benefit to the group.

The mammography recommendations, like the guidelines for back surgery issued by AHCPR 15 years earlier, involved replacing some uses of a technology with a more conservative approach. Health care providers and the public at large have an appetite for the new.[85] Calls for doing less can be more difficult to accept. Even so, recommendations to do less do not necessarily generate controversy. For example, there was little public debate in 1996 when the USPSTF recommended against the use of screening asymptomatic persons for lung cancer with either low-dose computerized tomography or chest X-ray. Breast cancer, however, has a far more powerful set of advocates than most other diseases,[86] and they mobilized to defend long-held positions on mammography screening.

Mammography and the Limited Focus of Breast Cancer Advocacy

The USPSTF's mammography guidelines had important economic implications for providers of the service in question—and indeed, there were some allegations that this was the primary source of the objections to the new guidelines. As one commentator put it, "The controversy is all about those billions of dollars that won't be flowing into the mammogram industry—the manufacturers, the hospitals, the clinics, the radiologists, the oncologists, the labs doing the biopsies, and so forth."[87] The conflict of interest between the economic interests of radiologists and the companies that manufacture mammography equipment, and the position of the American College of Radiology with regard to the USPSTF mammography recommendations, was noted by a 2010 article in the *Wall Street Journal*. "The American College of Radiology, a trade group, called the new government guidelines scientifically unfounded. . . . It received donations of at least $1 million each from GE Healthcare and Siemens AG. . . . Both companies make mammography equipment and MRI scanners."[88] The article also noted that Susan G. Komen, the leading breast cancer advocacy organization, also relied heavy on GE Healthcare for financial support.[89]

Beyond the obvious conflicts with radiologists and others with a financial stake in the use of mammography screening, several additional factors were at play in the screening controversy. One is the special nature of breast cancer, a disease that has generated a highly active advocacy community, many of whose members have long promoted screening mammography among

women 40 to 49 based on the presumption that early detection saves lives.
The research community has gone back and forth on the issue of screening
for years,[90] but this ambivalence had not always been reflected in the messages from the advocacy community. As one commentator put it, "Breast cancer is viewed as a plague. A 'war' on breast cancer is viewed as a crusade.
Screening mammography is Excalibur."[91] The USPSTF recommendations
differed from the longstanding public health message advanced by several
prominent advocacy groups, and they responded accordingly.

Susan G. Komen, along with its corporate partners, has been a dominant
voice in how the American public understands breast cancer, the value of
mammography screening, and the appropriate clinical and policy responses
to the disease.[92] In an effort to overcome the stigma of breast cancer, they
branded the disease as "pink."[93] The pink branding presents breast cancer as
"feminine, hopeful and uncontroversial"—and also focused efforts on individual rather than collective solutions.[94] Breast cancer has become big business, and there are millions of dollars at stake, not just for medical equipment
manufacturers and radiologists but for an array of corporations that have
become deeply involved in cause marketing around breast cancer.[95]

Both the Reagan and George H. W. Bush administrations called for reductions in government welfare spending and tried to emphasize the importance of corporate social responsibility as an alternative to government
programs.[96] The breast cancer movement built on this ideological approach
and encouraged corporations to align themselves with the movement. By
associating themselves with Susan G. Komen's "pink ribbon" campaign and
other efforts focused on mammography screening and research to develop
treatments, companies were able to enhance their reputations and increase
profits by donating money to a charitable cause.[97] The corporate involvement
in breast cancer has placed an emphasis on mammography screening that
ignores the limits of the technology and concerns about potential harms.[98]
The emphasis on mammography screening, despite decades of scientific
uncertainty about its value, has ignored potential environmental explanations for the disease. Smaller philanthropies, which want to emphasize
potential environmental causes or address racial inequalities in breast cancer, are unable to match these resources.[99]

The Limits and Politics of Weighting Risks

Another factor at play in the controversy was that the USPSTF based its
recommendation on a particular weighing of the evidence. In particular, how
much weight to give to false positives and the possibility that screening
might detect some cancers that would never become life-threatening were
central to the task force's recommendation. The USPSTF decided that the

risks of breast cancer screening of women under age 50 who carried no known special risk factors (for example, genetic factors) outweighed the benefits of screening. Some advocates of screening, reviewing the same evidence, reached the opposite conclusion.

Evidence about the value of health care technologies is not always subject to conflicting interpretations. For example, after years of hope and hype, the use of high-dose chemotherapy with bone marrow or stem cell transplantation for the treatment of advanced and early-stage breast cancer was stopped once there was sufficient evidence that this approach did not work.[100] Nevertheless, judgments about incommensurate factors will often be needed when evidence is evaluated. In response to the 2009 debate over mammography screening, Quanstrum and Hayward argued that it was important to acknowledge the value judgments at stake in the debate over the appropriateness of screening for women at different ages.

> What we often do not remember is that these thresholds—for example, an age of 40 versus 50 years or annual versus biennial routine mammography—are to some degree subjective and arbitrary. After all, scientific evidence can only help us describe the continuum of benefit versus harm. The assessment of whether the benefit is great enough to warrant the risk of harm—i.e., the decision of where the threshold for intervention should lie—is necessarily a value judgment.[101]

When conducting risk assessments or cost-benefit analyses, policy analysts often attempt to remain "value neutral" by assigning equal weights to different outcomes rather than weighting some more heavily than others. Adam Finkel argues that assigning equal weights to all outcomes is not value neutral and merely gives preferences to one set of value judgments over others. He calls for a more transparent process in which policymakers are explicit about their value assumptions.[102]

Obamacare, Rationing, and Hyperpartisanship

Perhaps the most important factor at play in the screening controversy was the highly charged political environment into which the USPSTF released its recommendations. Attacking the USPSTF and the mammography recommendations gave politicians an attractive way to advocate for women's health. The logic behind this is clear: if mammography screening is the key to reducing breast cancer mortality and breast cancer mortality is one of the leading causes of death among women, support for mammography screening is support for women's health, and an attack on mammography is an attack on women.

The recommendations also became part of the broader argument about the dangers of government control of health care. When the Obama administration had included $1.1 billion for comparative effectiveness research in the stimulus package in early 2009, opponents warned that such research would be used by government to ration care and deny patients lifesaving treatments. During a December 1, 2009 statement on the floor of the U.S. Senate, Senator Coburn (R-WY) claimed that seniors "are going to die sooner" as a result of health reform.[103] In fact, death rates due to breast cancer have continued to fall dramatically since the adoption of the American Cancer Society's recommendations,[104] but the hyperbolic prediction of Senator Coburn illustrates the dynamics of the debate over mammography screening, especially when it became entangled in the national health reform debate.

Although the USPSTF is independent, public and private health insurers often adopt its recommendations. In the context of the health reform debate, the recommendations were painted as a move toward government rationing of care and framed as "a glaring example of the dangers of increasing the Federal Government's control of health care."[105] An online editorial published by the *Wall Street Journal* argued that this was an example of the "political rationing of care" that we can expect under "ObamaCare."[106]

What opponents of the mammography screening recommendations were essentially saying was that research evidence of a technology's safety and effectiveness could be used by public and private payers to deny coverage for medical technologies. Provisions in the ACA were designed to prevent that outcome. Both the Senate's version of the ACA[107] and the final reconciliation act adopted by both houses of Congress "require qualified health plans to provide at a minimum coverage without cost-sharing for preventive services rated A or B by the U.S. Preventive Services Task Force,"[108] with amendments included in the Health Care and Education Reconciliation Act of 2010.[109] The USPSTF gave mammography screening for women age 40 to 49 a grade of C, so the charge that this recommendation could affect coverage was understandable. The ACA's provision does not explicitly state that recommendations with a grade below B should *not* be covered, but that is a reasonable interpretation of its intent. This helps to explain why HHS Secretary Sebelius made her statement about the recommendations and why Congress included a provision in the health reform bill to disregard them.

Conclusion

Professional and advocacy opposition, along with financial interests and ideological concerns about government "rationing," may create barriers to attempts to use findings from comparative effectiveness research and other clinical research studies to guide the use of preventive and treatment technologies, particularly when existing uses of those technologies are challenged. This seems particularly likely when health policy issues are highly salient to industry, professional, and consumer organizations.

With the adoption of the ACA and subsequent government-funded health insurance policies, health care costs will continue to be a major concern for policymakers. Both public and private health insurers will need to make difficult decisions about what services to pay for. Although analysts disagree about the potential for comparative effectiveness research to reduce health care spending,[110] the *idea* of using evidence to improve health care policy decisions enjoys support from a broad range of actors.[111] Nevertheless, the strong negative reaction to the USPSTF's 2009 mammography screening recommendations is a powerful signal that the *implementation* of comparative effectiveness research and evidence-based medicine can encounter great resistance, particularly when the evidence suggests that broadly accepted health care technologies that the health care community and patient advocates have promoted may not be worth the cost.

The USPSTF did not base its mammography recommendations on possible cost savings, but proponents of cost-effectiveness research and evidence-based medicine often claim that this research will reduce spending by eliminating unnecessary care.[112] The *reactions* to the mammography recommendations suggest that the health services research community needs to understand better what the public believes about evidence and ways that health care costs might be constrained.

The ACA called for establishment of a methodology committee to advise PCORI, which is charged with conducting comparative effectiveness research. The methodology committee is required to "develop and improve the science and methods of comparative clinical effectiveness research."[113] Establishing the credibility of its methods among a broad array of stakeholders will not insulate PCORI, or health services researchers more generally, from controversy. Nevertheless, establishing broader support for the value of health services research, coupled with sustained efforts to communicate more effectively with the public, is crucial as the United States grapples with how best to improve the quality and efficiency of its health system.

CHAPTER FOUR

When Medicare Said No for Amyloid PET Imaging

Medicare is a federal program that provides health insurance to three groups of beneficiaries: people age 65 years and older, people under age 65 with certain disabilities, and people regardless of age who have end-stage renal disease, defined as permanent kidney failure that requires dialysis or a kidney transplant. Although the Medicare program was expanded seven years after it came into existence to include beneficiaries other than people age 65 and older, its primary purpose is to provide health insurance for older Americans. Medicare Part A is hospital insurance that generally covers hospital care, skilled nursing facility care, hospice, and some home care services. Part B covers medical services, doctors and other health care providers' services, as well as outpatient care, durable medical equipment, home health care, and some preventive services. Medicare Part D provides prescription drug coverage, either from a Medicare Part D or a Medicare Advantage Plan.[1] Medicare Part D, which came into existence under the 2003 Medicare Modernization Act, extended coverage to outpatient prescription drug expenses, though it included a coverage gap—known as the "donut hole"—that temporarily limited coverage for drugs for some beneficiaries. Although the ACA closed the donut hole, the Act contained provisions that left Medicare beneficiaries susceptible to paying high out-of-pocket costs for medications.[2]

By the time the Medicare program reached its 50th anniversary in 2015, nearly all American families had come to rely on the program to pay for some of their aging relatives' medical expenses.[3] Because Medicare plays a significant role in enabling "the prowess of medicine to extend older lives, regardless of extent of disease, frailty, or age,"[4] technology developers, physicians, and patients have come to expect that Medicare will pay for new medical technologies or new uses of existing technologies to diagnose, prevent, and treat conditions and diseases that afflict older Americans.[5] Indeed, for much of its history, Medicare has had permissive coverage policies, paying physicians and hospitals with "few limits on reimbursable costs."[6] Yet the federal statute that created the Medicare program did not instruct Medicare to pay for all medical items and services for eligible beneficiaries. Instead, the statute prohibits coverage "for any expenses incurred for items or services which . . . are not reasonable and necessary for the diagnosis or treatment of illness or injury."[7]

In 2013, CMS—the agency that administers the Medicare program— ruled that it would not pay unconditionally for certain Medicare patients to undergo a brain imaging test known as *amyloid PET imaging*. The test involves using the radiopharmaceutical product florbetapir (Amyvid) with PET scan to determine whether patients have amyloid plaque in their brain, which are deposits of the protein fragment beta amyloid that builds up in the spaces between nerve cells.[8] Radiopharmaceuticals are radioactive drugs. PET uses a positron camera (tomography) to measure the decay of a radiopharmaceutical within human tissue, thus providing biochemical information about the tissue being investigated. It is used to evaluate normal tissue as well as diseased tissues associated with conditions such as cancer, ischemic heart disease, and several neurological disorders.[9]

When the FDA approved the use of florbetapir with PET imaging to identify amyloid plaque in living brain, the product developer—Eli Lilly and Company, along with many physicians, patients, and patient advocacy organizations such as the Alzheimer's Association—expected Medicare to pay for the test when physicians determined that it was "reasonable and necessary" for their Medicare patients. Yet CMS said it would only pay for amyloid PET imaging when relevant Medicare patients were enrolled in a clinical trial designed to determine whether information from the imaging test "potentially improves the participants' health outcomes."[10] The CED approach meant that CMS would be in the driver's seat for establishing what outcomes of interest in a relevant Medicare patient population it wanted to see as a condition of paying for amyloid PET imaging.

Imaging the Brain for Amyloid Plaque

Alzheimer's disease is a form of dementia, which itself is not a specific disease but a term for a "wide range of symptoms associated with a decline in memory or other thinking skills severe enough to reduce a person's ability to perform everyday activities."[11] Alzheimer's disease is said to account for 60 to 80 percent of all dementia cases.[12] In 2011, the National Institute on Aging (NIA) and the Alzheimer's Association proposed criteria and guidelines for diagnosing three stages of Alzheimer's disease: preclinical Alzheimer's disease, mild cognitive impairment due to Alzheimer's disease, and dementia due to Alzheimer's disease.[13] The preclinical diagnosis is "an 'at-risk state' defined by biomarkers and other risk factors, and uncoupled from clinical symptoms of the disease."[14] The proposed criteria and guidelines identified two categories of biomarkers (brain changes that indicate the presence or absence of Alzheimer's disease or the risk of developing the disease): changes in the level of amyloid plaque in a patient's brain and evidence of injured or degenerating neurons in the brain.[15]

Yet the presence of amyloid plaque in living brain does not mean that a person will develop Alzheimer's disease. For example, studies of autopsied brains have shown that approximately 33 percent of older individuals (20 to 65 percent, depending on age) who were cognitively normal had amyloid accumulation at levels consistent with the disease's pathology.[16] Moreover, amyloid plaque has been associated with other diseases such as dementia with Lewy bodies, cerebral amyloid angiopathy, Parkinson's disease, Huntington's disease, and inclusion body myositis.[17] Nonetheless, the ability to see amyloid plaque in living brain was welcomed as a major breakthrough for implementing the proposed criteria and guidelines the NIA and Alzheimer's Association developed for diagnosing Alzheimer's disease stages and for differentiating Alzheimer's disease form other dementias.

Asking for CMS Coverage

Within two months after receiving FDA approval for florbetapir, Lilly formally requested that CMS pay for amyloid PET imaging. The company was careful in describing the imaging tool as a "diagnostic test for the purpose of estimating beta-amyloid neuritic plaque density in adult patients with cognitive impairment who are being evaluated for Alzheimer's disease . . . and other causes of cognitive decline,"[18] rather than for the explicit purpose of diagnosing Alzheimer's disease. This was an important distinction, because in its approval letter to Avid Pharmaceuticals, the division of Lilly that developed florbetapir, the FDA said the following: "A positive Amyvid scan does not establish a diagnosis of AD or other cognitive disorder . . . safety and effectiveness of Amyvid have not been established for predicting development of dementia or other neurologic condition [and] monitoring responses to therapies."[19]

Lilly also asked CMS to reverse a national noncoverage decision the agency issued in 2000 regarding the use of PET imaging with radiopharmaceuticals for various neurologic conditions and other specific uses. In that decision, CMS had agreed on national coverage of PET with the radiopharmaceutical FDG (FDG PET) for either the differential diagnosis of frontal temporal dementia versus Alzheimer's disease when specific conditions were met. But for other uses, payment was conditioned on its use in a CMS-approved clinical trial that examined the clinical utility of FDG PET in diagnosing or treating dementing neurodegenerative diseases.[20] Others asked CMS to pay for amyloid PET imaging, including the Alzheimer's Association, a patient advocacy organization, and the Medical Imaging & Technology Alliance (MITA), which is a division of the National Electrical Manufacturers Association. MITA says its vision is for medical imaging to drive "effective patient care through screening, diagnosis and treatment," and that its mission is to "reduce regulatory barriers, establish standards, and advocate for the medical imaging industry." As of early 2018, the organization represented companies whose sales accounted for "more than 90 percent of the global market for advanced imaging technologies."[21]

CMS Decision-Making and Coverage Criteria

A comprehensive analysis of the Medicare program's decision-making pathways and of the evidentiary standards used in those pathways has yet to be written. However, health policy scholars point out that the fragmented decision-making process is due partly to statutory design and to decisions by CMS and its predecessor, the HCFA.[22] Private health insurers under contract with CMS make coverage decisions for prescription drugs.[23] The vast majority of coverage decisions for nonprescription technologies are made through the local coverage determination (LCD) pathway, which involves 12 Medicare Administrative Contractors (MACs) with jurisdiction over a specific geographic region. The coverage decisions each MAC makes apply only to the Medicare beneficiaries in the states in that MAC's region.[24] Because MACs are not required to follow the LCD outcome of other MACs, there is often variation across regions as to whether Medicare beneficiaries in a specific region obtain coverage for nonprescription medical technologies.

Coverage Criteria and the NCD Approach

When CMS is faced with a "big-ticket" technology or intervention that is "likely to have a significant impact on costs or quality of care, or those which are associated with safety concerns" the agency might use the national coverage determination (NCD) pathway, which accounts for roughly 10 percent of its coverage determinations.[25] A decision rendered through the NCD pathway takes precedence over decisions that MACs make via the LCD approach and applies nationwide.[26] Thus, how CMS defines "reasonable and necessary" when making coverage decisions using the NCD pathway has implications for the entire population of Medicare beneficiaries for whom a medical technology is available to diagnose or treat their condition.

HCFA struggled from the 1970s through the 1990s to establish formal rule-making criteria for "reasonable and necessary." The medical device industry initially pushed for such a rule then withdrew support when HFCA presented criteria requiring evidence of a technology's "medical benefit" and "added value."[27] Although HFCA never issued a final rule, the Medicare program's emphasis on relevant patient outcomes in its NCDs can be traced to the definition of medical benefit in HCFA's 2000 notice of intent for a proposed rule:

> We believe an item or service is medically beneficial it if produces a health outcome better than the natural course of illness or disease with customary medical management of symptoms. We would require the requester to demonstrate that an item or service is medically beneficial by objective clinical scientific evidence.[28]

In 2013, CMS updated its process for opening, deciding, or reconsidering NCDs. The agency reiterated that it reviews clinical evidence to determine whether an item or service "is reasonable and necessary for the diagnosis or treatment of illness or injury or to improve the functioning of a malformed body member for the affected Medicare beneficiary population" and noted that "FDA approval or clearance alone does not entitle that technology to Medicare coverage."[29] CMS typically issues about 10 to 15 NCDs a year,[30] with most resulting in a favorable coverage outcome, though CMS often attaches conditions on payment.[31] For example, of the NCDs for 56 FDA-approved medical devices issued between 1999 and 2011, Medicare agreed to pay for 75 percent of the devices, though coverage was generally more restrictive than what the FDA approved for market entry.[32]

The CED Pathway

In some instances when the outcome of the NCD is a denial of coverage, CMS says it will pay for the technology under the CED pathway. Although Medicare had previously attached conditions to payment for some technologies,[33] CMS formally initiated the CED pathway in 2004 under the leadership of Dr. Mark McClellan, an internist and economist President George W. Bush appointed to head the agency. McClellan had previously been the commissioner of the FDA. In the formal rollout of the CED pathway, McClellan said CMS was initiating a policy to close evidentiary gaps about the safety and effectiveness of medical technologies for Medicare beneficiaries. Dr. Sean Tunis, Medicare's chief medical officer, explained that the intent was not to force studies of every technology that Medicare paid for, but to use CED for "treatments that are potentially very important to the Medicare population but for which the evidence is not yet definitive." Given the growing federal budget deficit and looming health care costs, Tunis said that the United States had a choice: "Medicare could pay for everything, or we could develop a rational system to pay for the things that matter."[34] As of January 1, 2018, the CMS Web site listed 23 technologies it agreed to pay for under the CED pathway. Most are for medical devices. Four others involve the use of hematopoietic stem cells for transplantation, three involve some type of PET imaging, and one involves the off-label use of colorectal cancer drugs. For all but three of the 23 technologies, CMS has approved at least one clinical study and/or registry.

The NCD for Amyloid PET Imaging

CMS used the NCD process, which involved several steps over a two-year period, for making the amyloid PET decision. The agency initiated a 30-day public comment period regarding Lilly's request for coverage and then held a meeting of its Medicare Evidence Development and Coverage Advisory Committee (MEDCAC) to seek the "expert panel's input on whether the published evidence identified patient characteristics that would predict improved outcomes for patients who undergo" amyloid PET imaging.[35] MEDCAC (initially called the Medicare Coverage Advisory Committee) is an advisory committee created by HHS in 1998 to "review and evaluate medical literature, review technical assessments, and examine data and information on the effectiveness and appropriateness of medical items and services that are covered or eligible for coverage under Medicare."[36] Its role is to advise CMS when the agency undertakes a national coverage analysis of a medical technology. From 1999 through 2003, approximately 22 percent of CMS coverage analysis findings were based on evidence MEDCAC provided to the agency. Up to 100 members are appointed to MEDCAC, including patient advocates, consumer representatives, and industry representatives.[37]

CMS convened a panel of 12 MEDCAC voting members to address the issue of coverage for amyloid PET imaging. Formal presentations came from five invited guest speakers, "selected public comments" came from 11 physicians, and comments during the open public comment period came from one physician and one member of the lay public. Those giving a formal presentation included a leading Alzheimer's disease researcher, the chief medical officer of the division of Lilly that developed florbetapir, and the president of the Institute for Clinical and Economic Review, a nonprofit organization funded partially by health insurers and some pharmaceutical companies to conduct health technology assessments. At the end of the daylong meeting, 12 panel members voted on several questions CMS posed to them, with the key questing being "How confident are you that there is adequate evidence to determine whether or not PET imaging of brain beta amyloid changes health outcomes (improved, equivalent, or worsened) in patients who display early symptoms or signs of cognitive dysfunction?" The panel was instructed to use a one-to-five confidence scale. For low or no confidence, the score was one; for intermediate confidence, the score was three; and for high confidence, the score was five. The average score of the votes was 2.17: three members voted low or no confidence (1); five voted under the intermediate confidence level (2); three voted intermediate confidence (3); and one member voted between intermediate and high confidence (4).[38] Three months after the MEDCAC hearing, CMS opened a public comment period to receive responses to a proposed noncoverage decision it released for review.

Advocacy Positions Regarding Amyloid PET Coverage

While researchers were testing radiopharmaceuticals with PET imaging in clinical trials, and before Lilly received FDA market approval for florbetapir, leaders from companies developing radiopharmaceuticals and imaging devices; medical specialty groups such as the American College of Radiology and the American College of Radiology Imaging Network; physicians and researchers in the fields of radiology, neurology, and nuclear medicine; and patient advocacy organizations such as the Alzheimer's Association held workshops and published articles in which they advocated for Medicare coverage of amyloid PET imaging in the clinical setting under "appropriate use" criteria. They identified two primary justifications for their advocacy position: 1) that amyloid PET imaging was a breakthrough technology with value for a subset of cognitively impaired patients in specific clinical circumstances[39] and 2) that research endpoints for Medicare coverage of new PET radiopharmaceuticals should be intermediate outcomes such as positive change in patient management, rather than demonstration of a direct health benefit.[40]

In July 2011, a year before Lilly asked the FDA to approve florbetapir, MITA convened a workshop "to consider alternative pathways" for Medicare coverage policies that "might better encourage innovation and improve patient access to valuable new PET technologies."[41] Attendees at the workshop included leaders from imaging associations, other medical specialty groups, Lilly, patient advocacy organizations, health services researchers, radiologists, nuclear medicine physicians, cardiologists, and representatives from CMS. Workshop participants discussed CMS using the LCD process for PET radiopharmaceutical coverage decisions. They pointed out the LCD process was consistent with how the agency made coverage decisions for most new medical technologies, rather than the NCD pathway.[42] Left unstated was that the evidentiary standard for showing that a medical technology is "reasonable and necessary" has typically been lower in the LCD process than when CMS uses the NCD approach.[43] Other coverage options discussed at the workshop included a parallel review process, which involves concurrent FDA and CMS review of a medical technology to reduce the time between FDA approval and CMS review of requests for coverage.[44]

Importantly, workshop participants noted that coverage pathways other than the LCD process "may be rendered moot if the clinical evidentiary standards are unachievable."[45] They asserted that if "a diagnostic procedure is expected to demonstrate outcomes typically associated with therapeutic interventions, such as mortality reduction, such a standard would be unreasonable given the difficulty of demonstrating the impact of an imaging agent (and the imaging test performed with that agent) through a complex chain of diagnostic and therapeutic interventions to an ultimate patient outcome such as death."[46] For imaging technologies like PET, workshop participants contended that the focus should be on the change in therapeutic planning resulting from the diagnostic test, which "sometimes is a change to fewer medical interventions and perhaps to watchful waiting or palliative care."[47]

MITA held a second workshop in 2012 for the purpose of examining "which possible clinical research endpoints are appropriate evidentiary standards to demonstrate that new PET radiopharmaceuticals and new PET procedures lead to improved outcomes for Medicare beneficiaries" and thus should be paid for by CMS.[48] Among others at the workshop were two representatives from Lilly and two staff members from CMS. The workshop participants sent a clear message to CMS about coverage criteria for diagnostics like amyloid PET imaging. They contended that because diagnostics provide incremental benefit in therapeutic decision making, these technologies should be evaluated differently than therapeutic interventions, with emphasis on clinical evidence of the effect of the diagnostic on "intermediate endpoints, such as a beneficial change in clinical management (i.e., change in subsequent therapeutic or diagnostic interventions) that can be linked to improved health outcomes," and on "outcomes, or endpoints, appropriate to assessing whether diagnostic interventions are reasonable and necessary are best characterized as 'change in clinical management.'" They also asserted that the appropriate outcomes or endpoints are "distinct from the outcomes, or endpoints, classically applied in assessing whether therapeutic interventions are reasonable and necessary."[49]

Two weeks after CMS issued the proposed noncoverage decision, the Alzheimer's Association held its annual international conference, where many attendees lambasted the agency's preliminary decision to deny coverage for amyloid PET imaging. One clinician at the conference complained about "having our hands cuffed behind us as we try to help patients and their families is a moral dilemma,"[50] and another attendee said the proposed decision was "anti-moral" and "a disincentive to provide new technology to advance patient care."[51] Yet Susan Molchan, a physician who attended the conference, noted that some attendees "suggested that CMS was asking the right questions about the economics of health care and treating with appropriate seriousness the question of outcomes."[52]

Among others who supported CMS's noncoverage approach was Public Citizen, a consumer rights advocacy organization. In a letter submitted to CMS in response to the proposed noncoverage decision, Public Citizen noted that it was unaware of any completed, well-designed, controlled clinical trials that had evaluated whether information from amyloid PET imaging changed the health outcomes of any patient population.[53] And Robert Steinbrook, a physician and former member of MEDCAC, wrote in *JAMA Internal Medicine* that CMS's proposed decision agreeing to pay for amyloid PET imaging only under the CED pathway was a "courageous and innovative approach." Steinbrook said the CED approach "serves the public interest" and that CMS "would be irresponsible" if it paid for the test without adequate evidence of its role in Alzheimer's or other neurodegenerative diseases.[54]

The NCD Outcome

On September 27, 2013, CMS issued a final decision for noncoverage that included the CED option. A final NCD takes the form of a decision memo in which CMS summarizes its decision; describes the disease at issue and the background of the request for coverage; lists and summarizes the published literature and other evidence it reviewed regarding the technology's use and patient outcomes; responds to comments submitted during the public comment period(s); analyzes and discusses the evidentiary issues and relevant outcomes data; and explains its final decision. In addition to obtaining input from MEDCAC, CMS said that it reviewed a handful of position statements from several nuclear medicine and physician professional societies, as well as from disease advocacy organizations, as well as published studies involving the use of amyloid PET imaging with various patient populations and for various purposes.

CMS did not adopt the evidentiary framework that participants at the MITA workshops recommended for evaluating imaging technologies. Instead, the agency referred to an evidentiary framework that Mol et al. developed for evaluating a diagnostic technology. They said that the practical value of a diagnostic test necessitates taking into account subsequent health outcomes that result from the use of test information in guiding decisions to start, stop, or modify treatment.[55] CMS also referred to the five-level hierarchical framework Fryback and Thornbury developed for identifying evidence of improved patient outcomes.[56] In evaluating amyloid PET imaging, CMS applied levels two through five: the accuracy, sensitivity, and specificity of the diagnostic test (level two); whether a physician's diagnostic thinking changes as a result of the test information (level three); and the test information's effect on the patient management plan (level four) and patient outcomes (level five). CMS said it "generally found evidence of efficacy at level five more persuasive to support unconditional coverage" and that "coverage supported by that level or higher evidence results in the greatest benefit for Medicare beneficiaries."[57]

CMS pointed out that Medicare regulations require that for coverage, a diagnostic test must be ordered by the physician treating "a beneficiary for a specific medical problem" and who uses the results in the management of that specific problem. While it did not expect a diagnostic test to directly change patients' health outcomes, CMS said that it did expect a diagnostic test to affect health outcomes "through changes in disease management brought about by physician actions taken in response to test results."[58] Changes in disease management could include using or withholding a treatment, choosing one treatment over another, or choosing a different dose or duration of the same treatment, but CMS noted that data from amyloid PET imaging studies "are silent on health outcomes, and do not establish that the treating physicians appropriately base patient management on the PET test result." The agency also noted that most studies focused on test characteristics and did not consider health outcomes. "We believe," said CMS, that "health outcomes are more persuasive than test characteristics."[59] And to drive home the point one more time, CMS said, "there is no convincing evidence that the scan changes physician management of the patient in a meaningful manner (e.g., there is no convincing benefit to Medicare beneficiaries)."[60]

In response to the claim by some stakeholders of the "value in knowing" that a patient has amyloid plaque in his or her brain, CMS said there is an implicit, though incorrect, assumption that a positive scan means that a patient has Alzheimer's disease. The agency acknowledged that at some point, amyloid PET imaging might be used to establish a positive diagnosis of the disease in certain subpopulations, but that based on existing evidence, it could not "confidentially conclude that PET [amyloid] imaging improves health outcomes in beneficiaries who display signs or symptoms" of Alzheimer's disease.

CMS also addressed the issue about whether there was sufficient evidence of value to patient outcomes if an amyloid PET scan shows that a patient does not have amyloid plaque in his or her brain. The agency said that three questions were relevant in assessing the value of a negative scan. Could harm be avoided that would have otherwise occurred from a misdiagnosis of Alzheimer's disease, resulting in prescribed treatments for symptoms caused by other diseases? Could the quality and efficiency of clinical trials be improved to identify effective treatments for Alzheimer's disease? Could the clinical workup for other diseases that may be potentially treatable be expedited?

CMS acknowledged that there was promising evidence that information from amyloid PET imaging could change physician management of patients in a meaningful way and thus was willing to pay for one amyloid PET scan per patient who was enrolled in a clinical trial that addressed one or more aspects of three questions: Do patient health outcomes improve by using amyloid PET imaging results, with meaningful outcomes of interest including "avoidance of futile treatment or tests; improving, or slowing the decline of, quality of life; and survival?" Are specific subpopulations, patient characteristics, or differential diagnoses predictive of improved health outcomes in patients whose management amyloid PET imaging guides? Can improved health outcomes result from using amyloid PET imaging to guide patient management and to enrich clinical trials seeking better treatments or prevention strategies for [Alzheimer's disease], by selecting patients on the basis of biological as well as clinical and epidemiological factors?"[61]

Responses to the Final Decision

On the day CMS released its final decision, Lilly stated in a press release that the outcome "is not only contrary to expert opinion and published Appropriate Use Criteria previously recommended by the Alzheimer's Association and the Society of Nuclear Medicine and Molecular Imaging, but contradicts the statutory authority CMS has over coverage determinations for diagnostics." The agency, said Lilly, "is challenging the value of the only technology approved by the [FDA] for estimating beta-amyloid neuritic plaque density in the living brain, which can aid in helping doctors make a more informed diagnosis."[62]

Nearly a year after CMS issued its decision, three women—reportedly with funding from Lilly—filed a lawsuit against the agency.[63] They argued that because Medicare is required by law to pay for "reasonable and necessary" items and services, that the proposed CED pathway was an "unprecedented condition to coverage" and thus "fundamentally inconsistent with the plain language" of the Medicare statute.[64] The *Wall Street Journal* noted that financial analysts had estimated that with Medicare coverage for amyloid PET imaging, Lilly could have generated "perhaps $500 million in annual revenue." But without such coverage, the estimated annual revenue outlook was "maybe $100 million."[65]

In a memorandum opinion issued in July 2016, the U.S. District Court for the District of Columbia ruled that "the plain text of the Medicare Act did not preclude [CMS's] consideration of health outcomes and disease management in determining whether to afford coverage" for amyloid PET imaging as "reasonable and necessary for diagnosis."[66] However, the court also ruled that the "NCD did not adequately explain why that standard" differed from prior coverage outcomes resulting in CMS currently paying for amyloid PET imaging and FDG PET under certain conditions. The court determined that the agency's failure to "offer a sufficient rationale for treating these two tests differently" was arbitrary and capricious under the Administrative Procedure Act[67] and remanded the matter to CMS for further proceedings consistent with the memorandum opinion. Whether and how CMS has responded to the requirement for providing such a rationale is unclear.

The IDEAS Study

Although the Alzheimer's research community, the imaging device industry, and many physicians and patient advocacy organizations were unhappy with CMS's noncoverage decision, several of these stakeholders agreed to develop a clinical trial protocol to present to CMS for the CED pathway.[68] The Alzheimer's Association took the lead in this effort. The organization formed a research study team, and using an iterative process, obtained feedback "from a Scientific Advisory Board, an Industry Stakeholder group, and the CMS Coverage Analysis Group" in developing a research protocol. The outcome of the 18-month initiative was the "Imaging Dementia—Evidence for Amyloid Scanning (IDEAS) Study," an open-label, longitudinal cohort study that CMS approved in 2015 for its CED pathway.[69]

Sponsored by the Alzheimer's Association and managed by the American College of Radiology and the American College of Radiology Imaging Network, the IDEAS study is modeled after the largest successful CED study: the National Oncologic PET Registry (NOPR). Between May 2006 and April 2009, clinicians using PET submitted nearly 133,000 cases to the registry. Based on NOPR study results, CMS expanded PET coverage to several additional cancers and clinical indications.[70]

The CMS-approved study officially began on February 8, 2016, with the goal of enrolling 18,488 Medicare beneficiaries age 65 or older who met the study's eligibility criteria. The primary objective of Aim 1 is to determine whether the imaging test "will lead to a ≥ 30% change between *intended* and *actual* patient management within 90 days (75–105 day allowable range) in a composite measure of at least one" of three outcomes: drug therapy for Alzheimer's disease, other drug therapy, and counseling about safety and future planning.[71] For Aim 1, data will be collected for the first 11,050 participants enrolled in the study. Aim 2 of the study will use Medicare claims data to compare the medical outcomes at 12 months of the 18,488 participants in the longitudinal cohort who undergo amyloid PET imaging (amyloid PET-known), with a matched cohort of patients who never had the imaging test (amyloid PET-naïve). The primary objective is to determine if the testing in the amyloid PET-known cohort "is associated with a ≥ 10% reduction in hospitalizations and emergency room visits in comparison to the matched amyloid-PET naïve patients."[72] On December 6, 2017, the enrollment period was closed, and amyloid PET scans for all study participants were expected to be completed in January 2018.[73]

At the Alzheimer's Association's international conference in the summer of 2017, the study's investigators presented interim results from the "first 3,979 participants for whom case report forms were completed by participating dementia specialists both before and 90 days after the PET scans."[74] The median age of participants was 75 (range: 65–95); 64.4 percent had been diagnosed with MCI, and 35.6 percent met criteria for dementia. The interim results revealed changes in medical management in 67.8 percent of patients with mild cognitive impairment, with 47.8 percent of change involving drugs for Alzheimer's disease, 36.0 percent involving other drugs, and 15.3 percent related to counseling. The investigators also reported that information from amyloid PET scans "reduced the need for additional diagnostic testing such as neuropsychological testing (from 26.3 percent recommended pre-PET to 11.0 percent recommended post-PET) and spinal fluid testing (from 10.5 percent to 1.0 percent)."[75]

Conclusion

Since the late 1990s—in the midst of increasingly partisan debates over whether to expand benefits to Medicare patients, how to finance the program, and how to control medical costs,[76] CMS has gradually emphasized that to meet the statutory requirement of paying only for "reasonable and necessary" services, a physician's claim of "reasonable and necessary" may not be sufficient. Moreover, "over time and in fits and starts,"[77] the agency has embraced a wider perspective about safety and effectiveness than a narrow biomedical focus on intermediate or short-term end-points, emphasizing whether a technology "improves final outcomes of interest—such as functional status, quality of life, disability, major clinical events, and death—and whether it does so in typical patient populations."[78]

Nonetheless, even when CMS reviews a technology under the NCD pathway, it typically issues a favorable coverage decision. For instance, in 59 percent of the 213 NCDs the agency issued between 1999 and 2012, CMS agreed to pay for the technology.[79] Moreover, CMS tends to pay for FDA-approved devices more often than not.[80] Yet the agency does refuse to pay for some technologies, and the amyloid PET decision was consistent with the incremental approach CMS has taken for granting coverage for the use of PET scans in oncology and for dementia and neurodegenerative disease. For instance, of the 12 NCDs regarding the use PET imaging CMS issued between 2000 and 2009, the agency only agreed to pay for seven of the PET technologies when specific conditions were met.[81] Three indications for the use of PET imaging are listed on the agency's Web site as CED outcomes: FDG PET and other neuroimaging devices for dementia, NaF-PET for bone metastasis, and amyloid PET.

That CMS agreed to an open-label, longitudinal cohort design for the IDEAS study, rather than a randomized controlled design, suggests that the agency is not rigid in requiring that all outcomes evidence be generated from RCTs. Moreover, for Aim 1 (the assessment of amyloid PET information on patient management), the agency approved a composite measure of intended and actual change in patient management that involves one of three activities: use of an Alzheimer's drug, use of another drug therapy, and counseling about safety and future planning. Given that Congress has reined in the agency's ability to use cost-effectiveness[82] and comparative-effectiveness analysis in making coverage decisions in response to fears that findings will be used to restrict patients' access to care, weaken physicians' autonomy, result in health care rationing, and threaten biomedical innovation,[83] the amyloid PET decision can be viewed as a compromise approach to payer coverage. The IDEAS study will generate outcomes data that were not available to CMS when it conducted the NCD process, even if the data are not obtained from RCTs.

There is no guarantee, however, that CMS will agree to pay for a technology after reviewing results from a CED study. Indeed, few CED studies have led to a change in coverage policy.[84] Why such a change has not occurred is unclear, since no empirical analyses have been conducted of the 23 CED technologies listed on CMS's Web site. Kramer and Kesselheim point out that a barrier to coverage after implementing the CED approach is CMS's failure to provide criteria for what it considers convincing evidence for a favorable coverage decision. They offer several policy recommendations for developing and conducting CED studies: making protocols of CED studies publicly available, pooling study data from multiple sites for analysis and presentation, and developing a process for timely posting of study data. Based on information available from the IDEAS Web site, this CED study has several features that Kramer and Kesselheim recommended. The study is hypothesis driven; it specifies the primary and other endpoints; and the study protocol, data sharing, and publications policy are available on its Web site. Importantly, the IDEAS leadership team includes the chair and cochair of the NOPR, and these individuals also serve as investigators on the study.

Kramer and Kesselheim also recommend actions that CMS could take both for the NCD and CED models: provide more clarity about the level of evidence needed to meet the "reasonable and necessary" standard for the CED pathway, consider convening expert advisory panels for individual NCDs to address issues about study design, study endpoints, and evidentiary requirements of study data for showing the technology is "reasonable and necessary," and provide a hypothesis-driven description of the evidence needed to resolve the questions the study is designed to address. Others have suggested that Congress and the public should be involved in addressing coverage policy issues. For example, in response to HCFA's failed attempts from the 1970s through the 1990s to develop specific coverage criteria, Foote suggested turning to Congress. She contended that "[G]iven the pivotal role that new technologies and procedures play in health care, it is appropriate that the elected representatives grapple with these issues and be accountable for them."[85] And Muriel Gillick has suggested that "[A] debate in Congress over legislation to revise the 'reasonable and necessary' criteria would give the problem of determining Medicare coverage of new procedures and devices the public attention it deserves."[86]

Yet the evidence disputes we examined in this and other chapters suggest there may be no "institutional fix" for establishing evidentiary criteria for CMS coverage of medical technologies. If, as we contend, ideas about science, values about risks and benefits of technologies, and economic interests regarding innovation and market entry are at play in health technology assessment, then those forces will be at play regardless whether the arena of decision-making is Congress or an administrative or regulatory agency. The development and passage of the 21st Century Cures Act is a good example of how ideas, interests, and values are embedded and operate within all political institutions. Whether and how these forces will influence CMS decision making regarding coverage for amyloid PET imaging when the final results from the IDEAS study become available remains to be seen.

CHAPTER FIVE

Placing a Value on Cure: Lessons from the New Generation of Hepatitis C Drugs

On December 6, 2013, the FDA announced that it had approved a new drug for the treatment of hepatitis C, a common and potentially deadly virus. The drug, known as Sovaldi, was developed by Gilead Sciences and was hailed as a breakthrough in the treatment of the disease. The director of antimicrobial products at the FDA claimed that the approval of Sovaldi represented "a significant shift in the treatment paradigm for some patients with chronic hepatitis C."[1] Less than one year later, the FDA approved another drug from Gilead called Harvoni, that was even more effective and did not require patients to use other therapies. The excitement about the potential for these drugs to help people with hepatitis C was tempered by the high price of these treatments. The initial price for Sovaldi was $1,000 per pill—and Harvoni was even more expensive. The cost of these new medications, which were in great demand, threatened to place great strain on the U.S. health care financing system. Public and private payers responded by attempting to restrict access through a variety of policies, including efforts to limit coverage to patients who had already experienced advanced liver damage from the virus. Advocacy groups, physicians, and individual patients fought against these restrictions with some success.

Although the price of these drugs has fallen in recent years, concerns about the total cost of treating hepatitis C remain. More importantly, the case of these new treatments raises important questions about how to evaluate the value of expensive health care technologies. What evidence is relevant when making these decisions? How much value do we place on health improvements? What criteria should we use? The United States has struggled to answer these questions for medical technologies that offer small marginal benefits to patients. Ironically, evidence that a drug is highly effective does not make it any easier to develop answers. In some respects, the evidence of great effectiveness makes these conversations even harder.

Incidence and Consequences of Hepatitis C

What Is Hepatitis C?

Hepatitis C is a blood-borne viral infection that causes infection in the liver and interferes with the organ's ability to process blood, filter toxins from the body, and store glucose and vitamins. For about 20 percent of people who are infected with hepatitis C, the body's immune system will remove the virus without treatment. About 80 percent of those with the virus will develop a chronic infection that their immune systems will not remove. Furthermore, about 60 percent will develop chronic liver disease, and about 20 percent of those who are infected will develop a serious complication. These complications include decompensated cirrhosis (scarring of the liver) and hepatocellular carcinoma (liver cancer).[2] People with a chronic hepatitis C infection may experience symptoms that include nausea, vomiting, skin problems, blood disorders, and weight loss. Studies have found that people with hepatitis C are at increased risk for poor quality of health and death.[3] Every year, about 15,000 people, or between 1 and 5 percent of those infected, die from complications associated with hepatitis C.[4] Although the health consequences of hepatitis C can be deadly, the vast majority of people living with hepatitis C do not experience symptoms, though they can still infect others with the virus.[5]

Hepatitis C is both more common and more serious than hepatitis A or B. Hepatitis A can lead to nausea, abdominal pain, joint pain, fever, loss of appetite, and jaundice—and these symptoms may last for weeks. In the case of hepatitis A, however, the body's immune system will remove the virus, and it will not lead to a chronic infection. There is a vaccination that can prevent hepatitis A. Hepatitis B can lead to chronic infection and will do so in 90 percent of infants who contract the disease. This disease may result in anemia, kidney failure, cirrhosis, liver cancer, or liver failure. There is no cure for hepatitis B, and patients who develop severe problems may require a liver transplant. Fortunately, there is a vaccination for hepatitis B that can prevent the disease.[6] Hepatitis C is a bigger public health problem because it is even more likely to result in chronic infection than B, and there is no vaccine to prevent the disease. Therefore, the recent treatments that can eliminate the virus for most patients are an important development.

There are six different forms of the hepatitis C virus, and they are classified based on genotype (GT1–GT6). The different genotypes do not vary in their severity or their potential impact on the liver, but each responds differently to treatment. As a result, knowing the genotype of the infection helps clinicians identify appropriate treatments. In the United States, more than 75 percent of those infected with hepatitis C have GT1. Almost all the other people with hepatitis C have GT2 or GT3.[7]

How Many People Are Infected with Hepatitis C?

Most estimates suggest that between three and five million people in the United States are infected with hepatitis C—and there are an estimated 70 million people infected with the virus worldwide. The estimates vary because the rates of screening and diagnosis for hepatitis C are extraordinarily low. For many years, the failure to seek testing may have been reinforced by a lack of effective treatment.[8]

What Are the Characteristics of People Who Are Infected?

There appears to be a high rate of hepatitis C infection among the "baby boom" cohort of people born in the United States between 1945 and 1965. Studies of data from the National Health and Nutrition Examination Survey and the U.S. Department of Veterans Affairs indicate that three-quarters of baby boomers may be infected with hepatitis C,[9] an estimate that is emphasized in many of the direct-to-consumer marketing ads from Gilead, the producer of Sovaldi and Harvoni, two of the biggest-selling hepatitis C drugs.[10] The high concentration of the virus estimated among members of this cohort has led the Centers for Disease Control and Prevention (CDC) to recommended testing all individuals in this birth cohort. In 2013, the USPSTF gave this recommendation a grade of B, which means "there is high certainty that the net benefit is moderate or there is moderate certainty that the net benefit is moderate to substantial."[11]

Even though all baby boomers are at a high risk for being infected with hepatitis C, it is critical to recognize that the infection rate is higher among injection-drug users, the Medicaid population, and the prison population than among higher-income people with private health insurance.[12] The highest rates of hepatitis C infection are found among poor, uninsured, urban populations with poorer access to testing and treatment.[13] In addition to these groups, there may be higher rates of infection among people who immigrate to the United States from regions with high overall rates of hepatitis C. These include Egypt, Vietnam, and Eastern Europe.[14]

The demographic profile of the infected population is important for at least two reasons. First, it means that a large percentage of the population with hepatitis C is, or will be, eligible for government health insurance or health care programs, including Medicare, Medicaid, the prison health systems, and the Veterans Administration Health System. As a result, hepatitis C "has been called 'a disease of the marginalized' due to its disproportionately high prevalence among: the homeless (22%–53%), the severely mentally ill (19%), prisoners (23%–41%), and intravenous drug users (58%)."[15] The stigmatization of the population most closely associated with the virus may help to explain the policy response to it and raises questions about the politics of assigning a value to its detection and cure.[16] As Ingram and Schneider explain, the negative construction of a policy's target group as undeserving can be used to justify limited government spending on that group.[17] In the case of hepatitis C, it has contributed to a policy response to the price of treatment that is inconsistent with the responses of public and private payers to high-cost treatments for other diseases that are not as closely associated with these social groups.

Evolution of Hepatitis C Treatment

Until the 1990s, there was no treatment available for hepatitis C. In the early 1990s, researchers and clinicians discovered the benefits of interferon therapy, which involved injections three times each week and required a 24-to-48-week course of treatment.[18] In addition, the outcomes for most patients receiving this therapy were poor. By the end of the 1990s, treatment had improved, and the standard treatment for hepatitis C was pegylated interferon alpha and ribavirin. While this was more effective, this treatment was limited in several ways. First, this treatment had limited efficacy in hepatitis C patients with GT1, the most common form of the virus. Second, interferon alpha and ribavirin had significant side effects.[19] Interferon can lead to interferon-induced bone marrow depression, flulike symptoms, neuropsychiatric disorders, and autoimmune syndromes. Ribavirin, with which it is paired, can lead to hemolytic anemia, although this side effect can be reversed with additional treatment. In addition to the additional emotional and physical pain they caused patients,[20] these side effects also resulted in lower adherence, with 10 to 20 percent of patients failing to complete treatment.[21] For all patients with liver damage, treatment is expensive. For patients who ended up requiring a liver transplant, the costs were much greater. The estimated cost of a liver transplant in 2011 was $577,000.[22]

Since 2011 the FDA has approved several antiviral drugs for hepatitis C capable of eliminating detectable levels of the virus for many patients. The first few of these drugs were limited in their efficacy, but on December 6, 2013, Sovaldi, manufactured by Gilead, was approved for use by the FDA. Sovaldi is a once-a-day pill that must be used in combination with interferon and ribavirin, the previous treatments for hepatitis C, for patients with the most common form of hepatitis C, GT1. For patients with GT2 and 3, Sovaldi can be used in combination with ribavirin only. Clinical trials found that Sovaldi, in combination with these other therapies, was able to eliminate detectable levels of hepatitis C virus in the blood, what is known as "sustained virologic response" (SVR), at a much higher rate than previous treatments. Among patients with the GT1 version of hepatitis C, about 92 percent were able to achieve SVR in 12 weeks. Among patients with GT2-4, in which Sovaldi was combined with ribavirin, between 86 and 97 percent achieved SVR—and few patients stopped treatment as a result of side effects.[23] Following the approval of Sovaldi for the treatment of hepatitis C, Dr. John Ward, the director of the CDC's Division of Viral Hepatitis, expressed the enthusiasm shared by many when he announced, "Today marks a landmark advance in the treatment of hepatitis C, opening up new opportunities to stop the spread of this virus and the ravages of this disease."[24]

Less than one year later, on October 10, 2014, the FDA approved Gilead's Harvoni (ledipasvir and sofosbuvir), the first interferon-free direct-acting antiviral therapy for chronic hepatitis C virus GT1 infection. Unlike Sovaldi, Harvoni does not need to be taken in combination with ribavirin. Harvoni was approved as a breakthrough drug therapy. It was reviewed under the FDA's priority review program, which involves expedited review of drugs for serious conditions that would provide significant improvement in safety or effectiveness.[25]

Three clinical trials involving 1,518 participants evaluated the ability of Harvoni to achieve SVR. The participants in all three trials were randomly assigned to groups receiving Harvoni with ribavirin and those who received Harvoni without ribavirin. The first trial, which involved patients who had never been treated, found that 94 percent of those who received Harvoni for eight weeks and 96 percent of those who received Harvoni for 12 weeks achieved SVR. The second trial found that 99 percent of participants, with and without cirrhosis, who had not previously received treatment achieved SVR after 12 weeks. The third trial involved patients who had not responded to treatment and found that 94 percent of those who received Harvoni for 12 weeks and 99 percent of those who received Harvoni for 24 weeks achieved SVR. The inclusion of ribavirin did not improve the results in any of the trials.[26]

The consistent findings of such a high percentage of participants achieving SVR without the use of interferon or ribavirin was hailed as a breakthrough in the treatment of hepatitis C. In the popular media, however, the discussion about this advance in the treatment of hepatitis C was dwarfed by the reaction to the price of the new treatments. When Sovaldi was released, Gilead set the initial price at $1,000 per pill, for a total of $84,000 (plus the cost of interferon and ribavirin, which need to be taken with it) for a typical course of treatment. It was called the "poster child" for out-of-control drug prices. Gilead anticipated that there would be negative public reaction to this price. In an internal email, Gilead's executive vice president for commercial operations wrote, "Let's not fold to advocacy pressure in 2014 . . . Let's hold our position whatever competitors do or whatever the headlines."[27] When it released Harvoni, Gilead announced that the price would be even higher, at $1,125 per pill for a total cost of $94,500, although this was about the same as the cost of Sovaldi combined with the cost of the other treatments with which it must be used.

Public- and Private-Payer Coverage Policies

In response to the price, both public and private insurers have sought to limit the drug's availability.[28] To do so, public and private payers adopted a variety of strategies. Rather than remove the drugs from their formularies, several Medicaid programs and most commercial health insurance companies restricted access through prior authorization requirements. These included requiring that the drug could only be prescribed by specialists and by restricting access to people with advanced liver disease. Commercial health insurance companies were also able to restrict access by charging higher copayments for these drugs.[29]

The federal Medicaid law gives states broad discretion regarding prior-authorization criteria. A study of Medicaid restrictions on new treatments for hepatitis C found that 34 states had enacted regulations that restricted access to these drugs to patients who had experienced advanced liver disease, based on the level of scarring on the liver.[30] By the time these restrictions were challenged in court, the total number of states with such policies was 35. In addition, 37 states required patients to provide urine samples to check for alcohol and drug use and required a period of abstinence (usually six months) to receive treatment. The Medicaid programs in 29 states required a gastro-enterology, hepatology, infectious-disease, or living-transplant specialist to prescribe these drugs.[31] Finally, another policy that several states used was the "once in a lifetime" rule, which allows Medicaid programs to refuse coverage for anyone who became reinfected with the virus.[32]

Commercial insurer restrictions paralleled those enacted by many state Medicaid programs. However, private insurance companies and state-managed programs alike commonly employ similar coverage restrictions. A study by researchers at Yale University found that about 25 percent of patients with hepatitis C were denied coverage of Harvoni, and there were no differences in practice between public and private payers. Other reports suggest that the number of denials was much higher, with as many as 80 percent of patients denied treatment on the initial application for coverage.[33]

The prison population not only faces the greatest risk for hepatitis C, they face the most significant restrictions on access to these new treatments. Federal courts have determined that prisons can restrict care to prisoners if the decisions do not exhibit "a deliberate indifference to serious medical need."[34] This standard includes a right to health care without undue delay, but it is limited to "serious medical needs."[35] Under this standard, states are still using several mechanisms to restrict access to the new drugs. A comprehensive study of state prison health systems found that 41 states gave higher priority to patients with cirrhosis, 23 states gave priority to patients with chronic hepatitis C, and 12 states consider a patient's chance of reinfection.[36] It is possible, because of lawsuits from prisoners who have been denied access to treatment, that this situation may soon change. In 2017 three prisoners brought a class action suit against the Florida Department of Corrections. The U.S. District Court for the Northern District of Florida ruled that the state's prison system had not provided adequate treatment, and the Department of Corrections had to produce a new plan showing how it would comply with the court's order.[37]

Implications for Health Care Spending

The spending implications of these new hepatitis C drugs are striking. After several years of declines in inflation adjusted spending on drugs, there was an increase in 2014 that was due in part to the introduction of Sovaldi and Harvoni onto the market. These two drugs have the potential to substantially increase Medicaid spending in the United States and place considerable pressure on the budgets of prison health systems. Even after accounting for the fact that Medicaid programs were receiving a discount of more than 20 percent from Gilead, many states argued that they had to use these other mechanisms to limit access.[38] The National Association of Medicaid Directors voiced its concerns to congressional leaders:

> Simply put, the federal Medicaid statute is not designed to allow states to respond to this new pricing approach for pharmaceuticals. Sovaldi is just the first of many such exceptionally high-cost "curative" specialty drugs. As more of the specialty drugs that are brought to market adopt this same pricing rationale, new thinking and approaches are required to safeguard the financial integrity of state Medicaid programs and ensure low-income patients can access appropriate medical innovations.[39]

A study published in the *Annals of Internal Medicine* estimated that if everyone who could benefit from the new therapies received them, public and private payers would need to spend $136 billion between 2014 and 2018 to cover the cost of treatment for hepatitis C patients. Just under half this total, $61 billion, would be the responsibility of public programs.[40] Even before the introduction of Harvoni on the market, the Kaiser Family Foundation did an analysis of the cost implications to the Medicare program of possible spending on Sovaldi and concluded that the cost implications for the federal government and individual beneficiaries would be significant. They argued that "if only 30 percent of hepatitis C-infected Medicare enrollees were treated with Sovaldi over the next two years, program costs would increase by $6.5 billion, and premiums and outlays for all Part D (prescription drug plan) enrollees would rise by 8 percent."[41] The implications for the prison health system are even more dramatic. The medical director of Oregon's state prison system claimed that the cost of treating all the system's prisoners who had the disease would cost four times the entire annual health care budget. He argued that paying to treat hepatitis C with these new drugs would make it impossible, without a massive expansion to the prison health system budget, to provide any other form of health care.[42]

The Advocacy Campaign for Expanded Access

One of the arguments frequently used by Medicaid directors and commercial insurers to defend restrictions on Sovaldi and Harvoni was that there is insufficient evidence to predict which patients infected with hepatitis C will develop liver disease. Considering the high price of these drugs, they reasoned that it does not make sense to treat all patients diagnosed with hepatitis C, because the majority will never develop clinical symptoms. Restricting access to patients with advanced liver disease helps to ensure that those with the greatest need are being treated. Medicaid directors did not invoke the idea of cost-effectiveness because public payers are not allowed to consider this when making coverage decisions, but commercial health insurers also argued that it would not be cost-effective to treat patients who would never develop liver problems with such expensive drugs.

The American Association for the Study of Liver Disease and the Infectious Diseases Society of America, two leading scientific associations made up of clinicians and scientists, both rejected these arguments. These associations, along with dozens of other advocacy organizations, argued that all patients with hepatitis C should have access to drugs that could achieve SVR. First, waiting until patients develop advanced liver disease increases the risk that patients will develop liver cancer. As several physicians have argued, the new hepatitis C drugs can eliminate the virus from a person's body, but they cannot undo liver damage.[43]

A second critique is based on a public health perspective. From this perspective, restrictions on treatment are a problem because asymptomatic individuals with the virus are still capable of infecting others.[44] We know that only about 20 percent of patients who are infected with hepatitis C will develop advanced liver disease, but we know less about how to predict whether this will happen for an individual patient. Even if an individual with the virus will not experience clinical symptoms, he or she will still be infected and could pass this along to other people. Because a large portion of patients are infected by sharing needles and other equipment to inject drugs, there is a significant risk of spreading the infection among drug users, but it is also possible to spread the virus more broadly through any contact in which people are exposed to infected blood. This can include sharing personal care items like razors or toothbrushes—and it can also be spread by having sexual contact.[45] Treatments that can eliminate a virus from an infected person are what economists called "mixed goods" because in addition to providing a benefit to the patient who received the treatment, they also generate external benefits for other identifiable groups.[46] If the goal of coverage policy is to improve the health of an entire population rather than to focus on the health of a particular individual, providing broader access to treatment makes sense. The logic is identical to the recommendations of UNAIDS for ending the AIDS epidemic. This plan calls for expanding testing so that 90 percent of all people living with HIV know their HIV status, 90 percent of all people diagnosed with HIV infection receive sustained antiretroviral therapy, and 90 percent of people receiving treatment achieve viral suppression. Models suggest that if these goals are achieved by 2020, HIV could be eradicated by 2030.[47] There are obviously many barriers to achieving this goal, but eliminating this disease is a possibility, and the new generation of therapies makes this a possibility for hepatitis C as well.

Nevertheless, because the lack of evidence about disease progression was part of the rationale for limiting coverage to those who had not developed advanced disease, PCORI held a stakeholder meeting in 2014 at which they decided to fund a comparative-effectiveness study to investigate whether treatment at various stages of liver fibrosis is equally protective against progression to advanced liver disease. Patients and clinician stakeholders at the meeting expressed concern that sponsoring a three- to four-year randomized trial could serve to delay the spread of insurance coverage for treating early-stage disease. Others expressed concern that since some insurers had started paying for Harvoni at diagnosis—in some cases because of patient litigation—institutional review boards that review and approve research with human subjects might balk at approving a study, and patients might be unwilling to enroll in one if insurers were already paying for the drug. In response to similar objections at a subsequent stakeholder meeting in 2016, PCORI reversed its decision and decided not to pursue this research.[48]

A Response to Stigmatized Patients?

An argument offered by advocates for expanded coverage is that the adoption of restrictive policies for the treatment of hepatitis C reflects the stigmatization of these patients. Hepatitis C patients are disproportionately poor and more likely to be prisoners and/or use injection drugs. Opponents of the policies that restrict access argue that the policies regarding payer coverage of Sovaldi and Harvoni stand in contrast to their coverage of very expensive cancer drugs, many of which are less effective. They argue that this is evidence that attitudes about the patients receiving these treatments is shaping policy. Because hepatitis C is prevalent among stigmatized groups that are often thought to be less deserving of public support,[49] payers are responding to the high price by enacting restrictions on use. Lynn Taylor, an infectious-disease physician in Rhode Island, articulated this position when she argued, "We don't withhold cancer treatment to only those with the most advanced stages of the disease. . . . We don't deny smokers treatment for lung cancer."[50] While few cancer drugs are as expensive on a per-pill or per-treatment basis, it is not uncommon for cancer treatments to cost $100,000 per year or more.[51] Public and private payers routinely cover these cancer therapies, even though they may not provide a cure but rather extend the lives of people living with metastatic disease. Robert Greenwald, the director of Harvard Law School's Center for Health Law and Policy Innovation, which played a lead role in many of the class action lawsuits against states that adopted restrictive Medicaid policies, agrees with this argument. He claimed that policies used to restrict treatment for hepatitis C would not be tolerated for other diseases, and this only occurs because hepatitis C patients are vulnerable and stigmatized.[52]

Role of the Courts

Along with mounting advocacy campaigns to pressure public and private payers to change their policies, several patients and advocacy groups started to pursue legal remedies. Several groups filed lawsuits against commercial insurers and Medicaid programs that had enacted restrictive policies. The American Civil Liberties Union, Harvard Law School's Center for Health Law and Policy Innovation, and prisoner rights organizations were all instrumental in helping advocates to file class action lawsuits in multiple states. In addition, the Massachusetts attorney general threatened Gilead with an investigation of its possible "unfair trade practice in violation of Massachusetts law," based on its pricing of Sovaldi and Harvoni.[53]

The plaintiffs in these cases argued that state Medicaid programs were violating the law by enacting restrictions on these drugs because Medicaid is supposed to cover medications if they are medically necessary.[54] They also argued that states would save money by providing these treatments, because the cost of treating people who become sick is even greater. Even before the courts decided these cases, the lawsuits began to have an impact on state policies. About a dozen states began to make it easier for patients to qualify for coverage. For example, many Medicaid programs began approving coverage for Harvoni, regardless of disease severity.[55] In 2014, 91 percent of states limited patient access to the new drugs to those with significant liver damage or a high fibrosis score, but by the end of 2017, only 46 percent of states were continuing to do so.[56] In 2017, that number has dwindled to 23 percent. When Pennsylvania lifted its restrictions, the state Medicaid office claimed that the policy change would present a "significant fiscal challenge."[57]

Price Negotiation and Competition

State Medicaid programs and commercial insurers have also been backing away from their initial restrictions on treatment because the prices of these drugs have fallen. At least two developments have contributed to the reduction in price. First, the FDA has started to approve newer and slightly less expensive competitors. As new entrants are approved by the FDA, it seems likely that the cost will come down further.[58] For example, Mavyret, a drug that can cure all six genetic types of hepatitis C, costs $26,400, which is significantly less than the discounted rates for Harvoni.[59] There are other drugs in the pipeline that may offer similar cure rates with shorter treatment periods and even lower costs.[60]

Second, Express Scripts, one of the largest pharmacy benefit companies in the United States, dropped Harvoni from its formulary. The move by Express Scripts prompted Gilead to begin negotiations to make sure their drugs were covered by formularies used by commercial health insurers. In 2015, Gilead negotiated five deals with commercial insurers by offering discounts of 46 percent for Sovaldi and Harvoni.[61]

Lessons from the New Generation of Hepatitis C Drugs

The reductions in the cost of the new generation of hepatitis C drugs does not eliminate the financial problems these drugs represent for state Medicaid and prison health systems. Even the reduced prices for Sovaldi and Harvoni—and the lower prices for more recent alternatives—are high and will place strain on the limited budgets of these programs. Equally important, it is likely that pharmaceutical companies will produce, and the FDA will approve, other expensive and highly effective drugs in the coming years. One example is Kymriah by Novartis, a treatment made by genetically reengineering a patient's white blood cells, which are later infused into the patient to identify and kill the cancer cells in the bloodstream. This cost of this new treatment, for a one-time infusion, will be $475,000. This price of Kymriah has led to alarm, not only about the implications for health care spending, but about whether it will be available to people who need it.[62] Researchers are hoping to develop similar therapies for solid cancers as well.[63] If they are successful, these drugs may be priced at similar levels.

The discussion of new hepatitis C drugs raises the larger question about drug prices in the United States. As with prices for other medical services, the United States has the highest prescription drug prices in the world. In his first State of the Union address, President Donald Trump focused on this issue. He stated that he wanted his administration "to make fixing the injustice of high drug prices one of our top priorities. Prices will come down," though he was not specific about how he would achieve this goal.[64]

When confronted with the high price of drugs in the United States, the pharmaceutical industry is quick to point out that spending on drugs represents only 10 percent of total spending in the United States. But the price of drugs in the United States is significantly higher than other countries and has been rising sharply since 2013. One study found that, among widely used inpatient pharmaceuticals, the U.S. prices are twice as high as those in Australia, Canada, and the United Kingdom.[65] Higher drug prices, combined with high rates of use, lead to drug spending in the United States that is more than double that in other high-income countries. In 2012, for example, the United States spent US$ PPP (purchasing power parity) 1,010 on pharmaceuticals per capita, compared with an average per capita expenditure in member countries of the Organisation for Economic Co-operation and Development of US$ PPP 498.[66]

Governments grant monopolies to drug companies in the form of exclusivity—certain delays and prohibitions on approval of competitor drugs, when the FDA approves a new compound. During the time when they enjoy these monopolies in the United States, they often raise the prices of the drugs repeatedly. Schering-Plough, for example, increased the price of Claritin 13 times during a five-year period. The company justified the increases because they said it would allow them to invest in research and development.[67] The combination of population aging; the growth of chronic illness; and the advent of new, highly effective, but extraordinarily expensive drugs raises fears about the implications of drug costs on health care spending and the economy.

Drug Company Responses to Price Complaints

The responses of Gilead to criticisms about the price of Sovaldi and Harvoni were similar to the arguments used by all pharmaceutical companies to justify high drug prices in the United States. Along with the need to recover their substantial investment in drug development, Gilead focused on the relative cost and effectiveness of their new drugs compared with existing treatments. Gilead has consistently said that its hepatitis C drugs are worth the price because of their effectiveness. According to a spokesman, "Gilead responsibly and thoughtfully priced Sovaldi and Harvoni."[68] Three years after the public outcry at the initial price of Sovaldi, the CEO of Gilead, John Milligan, expressed regret that the company had not been more responsive to the cost concerns, but continued to defend the underlying logic used by the company to set the price and continued to assert that, even at the high price, the drug represented a "good value."

> Yeah, it was an interesting launch for the HCV product. We priced the product at exactly the same as the existing standard of care, which worked about 50% of the time, and are providing a benefit that, based on real world experience, works about 98% of the time. From our perspective, it was a very good value. What happened was a failure to understand exactly how many people were direly ill and had to come into care. That is, there were hundreds of thousands of people who needed this immediately, whose doctors felt that they needed this immediately. The surge into the system was very large, and that created a lot of anxiety around the payers and of course created an outcry against us for having mispriced the product.[69]

The logic articulated by Gilead is not unique. Drug companies frequently justify the price of their products by arguing that they reduce spending on other medical interventions that would be required to treat people if they fail to take the drugs.[70] One obvious problem with this logic is the assumption that the price of alternative treatments is appropriate. Critics of the U.S. health care system argue that prices for all treatments in the United States are too high because we do not adequately negotiate prices with health care providers, drug companies, or medical device manufacturers.[71] The claim that a high-priced drug is a "good value" because it is less expensive than other treatments that are also overpriced is a curious position.

Another problem with this logic, from the perspective of a commercial insurance company or even from an individual Medicaid or prison health system, is that even if the claim is correct, the insurer who pays for the drug treatment may not be the one that benefits from the savings. When a payer refuses to cover a drug that may defer other spending, they are "hoping the patient will die on somebody else's dime."[72]

Even if we adopted a universal health care system based on social insurance principles in which the entire population was in a single risk pool, the argument would still be challenged because the evidence does not often support the claim that the spending on a drug or combination of drugs actually "saves" money. For example, one analysis of the new hepatitis C drugs showed that the drug would cost an additional $65 billion, but this would only reduce other health care spending by about \$16 billion.[73] The calculation is likely to depend on several factors, including what is included in the list of future costs and benefits. If we should include potential "downstream" costs and benefits associated with the use of a drug or other intervention, which downstream costs and benefits should be included in the analysis? Should it, as Meltzer and Magnus suggest, account for the costs and benefits of "unrelated illness and non-health care consumption and production during added life years?"[74]

How to Evaluate Value in the Context of Cure?

In the United States, critics often point to the unwillingness to make difficult choices about expensive treatments that offer little or small marginal benefit. Congress, for example, explicitly forbids the Medicare or Medicaid programs from making coverage decisions based on incremental cost-effectiveness.[75] This becomes an even more challenging question when there is strong evidence that a treatment offers a significant health benefit—or even a cure—as in the case of Sovaldi and Harvoni.

How should we place a value of the health benefit of a drug or other therapy? Economists often do so by first measuring the benefits of the drug in terms of health units. In Australia, New Zealand, and the United Kingdom, for example, they try to measure the number of QALYs produced by a drug. To calculate how much each of the gains in a QALY is worth, health economists remind us that people routinely place a price on securing themselves against illness or injury when they make decisions in the marketplace. For example, people make judgments about how much they are willing to pay for safety equipment. When making these choices, people are placing an implicit price on their risk of mortality. Economists have conducted studies looking at labor market data to estimate how much people are willing to pay to reduce the risk of mortality. If a person (or people in a particular country, based on a population study) are willing to forgo \$100 to reduce the risk of mortality by 1/1000, this gives a value of life of \$100,000 in the sense that the risk reduction is achieved in a population of 1,000: if mortality risk is reduced by 1/1000 per capita over a population of 1,000, this is the same as saying that we expect—statistically—one life to be saved in this population.[76] This appears to provide a useful way of placing a value on drugs and other therapies that offer dramatic improvements in health—but they face serous limitations. Even if we accept this approach to placing a price on reducing the risk of mortality, it is incredibly hard to come up with a reasonable estimate of the "willingness to pay" for a particular population. Studies that have attempted to do so produce estimates that vary widely.[77]

Another important critique of the standard economic approach to determining an appropriate price for drugs and other interventions is that the willingness-to-pay estimates do not adequately capture the opportunity costs associated with this spending. When countries evaluate the cost-effectiveness of new drugs, they compare the incremental gains in spending on a new treatment for a disease compared with existing treatments. This is helpful information, but it does not tell you what the return on spending additional money on the new drug is, compared with spending on some other socially useful good. Even if the only outcome that society values is good health, which seems unlikely, we should care about the impact of health care spending on our ability to pay for decent housing, high-quality education, and environmental protection, among other things. An incremental cost-effectiveness study that only compares choices among spending on different health care therapies cannot tell us about these other tradeoffs. For drugs like Sovaldi and Harvoni, which have high price tags and could benefit many people, the opportunity costs can be substantial. This can become a serious problem if the concept of "value for money" is offered as an antidote to cost worries.[78] Up-front investments in health care may be valuable in the long run but may simply not be affordable. A study by the New England Healthcare Institute on comparative-effectiveness research (with pharmaceuticals particularly in mind), makes a plausible case for innovation as a medical and economic value.[79] The implicit message is, yes, we know there is a cost problem, but we provide such a great return on investment, you should look to save money by cutting back on something else. It is a kind of elegant not-in-my-backyard defense. Unfortunately, the siren song of eventual payoffs does not address the problem of limited resources and fails entirely to take seriously the problem of opportunity costs.

Loss of Innovation

Another classic argument used to justify high drug prices is that they provide appropriate incentive for drug companies to pursue innovation. If the United States negotiated prices more aggressively, there would be a net loss to society because companies would no longer invest in the research and development necessary to produce the next "breakthrough" drug that dramatically improves treatment. This claim is based in part on the assertion that the cost of developing new therapies is large and requires "adequate" compensation.

Critics of the pharmaceutical industry often question how much drug development costs, and others raise questions about how much compensation is really justified. Arno and Davis, for example, point to 10 years of NIH funding for research "seeking nucleosides or nucleotide blockers precisely like Sovaldi for hepatitis C as evidence that a large share of the research that made it possible for Gilead to develop these drugs was paid for with tax dollars."[80] Furthermore, they point out that the publicly funded research was financed at a time when there was still enormous risk that the research would not bear fruit. Large pharmaceutical companies typically get involved in further research and development only after the publicly funded research, often conducted by smaller pharmaceutical companies, demonstrates a high probability of success. At that point, large pharmaceutical companies will purchase these smaller companies and the rights to all the compounds they have developed. This is exactly what happened in the case of Sovaldi.[81]

Uwe Reinhardt argued that, thanks to public investment in research and development, along with the government's patent laws, pharmaceutical companies should be thought of

> as fragile little birds that the protective hand of government carefully shields from the harsh vagaries of truly free, competitive markets. That protective hand consists of patents granted these producers by the US Patent and Trademark Office and market exclusivity that can be granted by the US Food and Drug Administration on request. It also consists of prohibiting resale of these products among customers, such as reimporting drugs from countries that have been granted lower prices.[82]

Under these circumstances, Reinhardt, Arno, Davis, and other critics of existing policy argue that the government should step in and protect American patients and other taxpayers from high drug prices. The Bayh-Dole Act allows the U.S. government to make drugs that were developed, in whole or in part with federal funds, available to patients on "reasonable terms." The act does not define what "reasonable" means, but Congress has never allowed public payers to step in and negotiate these terms.[83]

Conclusion

The case of new-generation hepatitis C treatments offers insights into the broader challenges facing the U.S. health care system. The United States has never adopted policies that place limitations on aggregate health care spending. At the same time, we have adopted policies that encourage the continual development of new health care technologies and limit the ability of government payers to negotiate the price of these technologies. Drug companies reinforce this perspective by pointing to economic evaluations that support the claim that many of their products offer a good return on investment. Although this claim may be in dispute for some drugs that offer small marginal improvements in health, evidence about the value of treatments that are capable of curing a disease are compelling. Good value, however, does not mean less expensive—and many new treatments have remarkably high prices. In the face of such cost pressures, payers in the United States often respond by passing costs along to individual patients, sometimes by restricting coverage. In the case of Sovaldi and Harvoni, this is precisely how public and private payers responded to these drugs. Advocacy efforts, including the use of class action lawsuits, helped to lift restrictions on coverage, but this does not address the cost problem these and other new, expensive drugs present. Unless policymakers are willing to have a difficult debate about how to address the opportunity costs associated with this spending, there is likely to be a continual battle between physicians, patients, and advocacy groups who expect public and private insurers to pay for patients' access to new therapies and insurers who limit such access.

CHAPTER SIX

Avastin and the Politics of Accelerated Approval

In 2008 the FDA approved the cancer drug bevacizumab, known as Avastin, in combination with paclitaxel (Taxol) to treat women with metastatic HER2-negative breast cancer who had not yet received chemotherapy for metastatic breast cancer. The approval was based on limited evidence about the drug's benefits and was approved under the agency's accelerated approval pathway. By 2011, following a year of heated debate, the FDA took the unusual step of revoking its approval for the use of Avastin for the breast cancer indication. In many respects, the FDA decision is an atypical case. Even though the number of drugs that have been approved through the FDA's expedited programs—including the accelerated approval pathway—has increased over the past two decades,[1] there are only a few examples in which the agency has acted to withdraw these approvals.[2] This exceptional case, however, offers insights into the potential concerns about recent efforts to make the FDA approval process faster by bringing drugs to market on the basis of even less evidence than has been required in the past. In light of the desire by many members of Congress and the Trump administration to make new drugs available on the market faster than ever, the lessons from the Avastin case are particularly salient.

Interest group politics are clearly important when it comes to the question of drug regulation standards. There are billions of dollars at stake with each decision, and the profitability of pharmaceutical companies is influenced by how many of their products make it to market and how quickly the FDA grants market approval. The actual cost of drug development is hotly debated,[3] but even lower-end estimates suggest that it costs several hundred million dollars to develop a new cancer drug.[4] Genentech, the company that manufactures Avastin, aggressively promoted to oncologists the "off-label use" of the drug for breast cancer in the years before the FDA approved it for the metastatic breast cancer indication. Particularly in treating cancer, physicians often prescribe drugs off label, meaning that they use the drugs to treat conditions other than those for which they were approved by the FDA. Although public and private health insurers sometimes pay for drugs prescribed off label, they often refuse to do so on the grounds that there is insufficient evidence of safety and effectiveness for off-label use and refer to the drugs as "experimental" or "investigational." Payers are more likely to reimburse for prescriptions when they are used for indications approved by the FDA and, as was the case with Avastin, less likely to do so if FDA approval for an indication has been removed.[5]

Fear that health insurance companies might refuse to pay for off-label use of Avastin if the FDA withdrew market approval for the breast cancer indication helped to drive the opposition to the FDA's decision. The financial implications of the agency's decisions to withdraw market approval for drugs is also important to the government, even though the FDA is not allowed to consider costs when it makes its regulatory decisions. As Dr. Eric Winer, the director of the Breast Oncology Center at the Dana Farber Cancer Institute, explained in reference to the Avastin decision, "it's hard to talk about Avastin without talking about costs. For better or worse, Avastin has become in many ways the poster child of high-priced anti-cancer drugs."[6] The accelerated approval process has become a mechanism for getting many high-priced drugs to market, and this has contributed to increased spending by public and private payers.

Physicians, patients, and patient advocacy groups also have a large stake in this debate. Neither physicians nor patient groups are always in favor of faster approval, but specialists and disease-specific advocacy groups often push for this because they hope to offer patients more options for treatment, with the possibility of life extension and the alleviation of suffering. In the case of Avastin, the physician and advocacy communities were divided, but opponents of the FDA's decision to withdraw approval for this indication were organized and vocal in their opposition, leading to a yearlong fight before the FDA made its final decision.

Questions about the speed of drug approval are usually caught up in partisan debates about the role of government. For example, Republican members of Congress often complain about the "red tape" of public bureaucracies. In 2014, Former House speaker and candidate for the Republican nomination for president, Newt Gingrich, called for eliminating the FDA because it is an "obsolete bureaucracy with obsolete rules that do more harm than good."[7] Former speaker Gingrich, like many other Republicans, has argued that allowing drugs to reach the market while they are still being tested would spur competition, lower drug costs, and get therapies to people who need them much earlier. President Trump, as a candidate in 2016, joined the chorus of people who criticized the FDA for slowing the adoption of "life-saving" drugs. After he was elected, he repeated these charges, arguing that agency requirements for approval were "slow and burdensome" and "keeps too many advances . . . from reaching those in need."[8] Under the direction of Scott Gottlieb, President Trump's director of the FDA, the agency has made several changes in policy designed to speed up the drug approval process by lowering evidentiary standards.[9] For example, in July 2017 the FDA announced that, when seeking approval to use a drug for a rare disease, companies could rely on data from previous clinical trials rather than conducting additional research.[10]

The Avastin experience raises questions about proposals to further speed the approval of new therapies. What does this case suggest for efforts by the Trump administration to further reduce the evidence required for accelerated approval? Does the Avastin case suggest that this policy change is dangerous because it could lead to the approval of drugs that do more harm than good—or does the Avastin case provide evidence that the accelerated approval approach should be expanded because the FDA is willing to act on new evidence and make difficult decisions about the use of popular treatments?

The Challenge of Treating Advanced Breast Cancer

Metastatic breast cancer is incurable, so the goals of treatment are palliation of symptoms and improvements in overall survival time. As with cancer more generally, breast cancer is more than one disease, and particular forms of cancer are more aggressive than others. Some forms of breast cancer are not responsive to hormone therapy, and many patients do not respond well to more traditional chemotherapies, but the frequency of recurrence has been reduced in recent years due to the development of new targeted treatments. Avastin is an example of a targeted therapy.

Avastin was developed in 2004 by Genentech and was used originally to treat metastatic colorectal cancer in patients for whom standard treatments were unsuccessful. Avastin was the first drug designed to block blood flow to tumors, an approach that was considered a breakthrough in the treatment of cancers. Cancer cells need blood for food and oxygen and to remove waste. Tumors can only grow beyond a few millimeters if they first grow additional blood vessels to feed the tumor. The growth of new blood vessels is a process called angiogenesis. Antiangiogenic drugs are treatments that stop tumors from growing their own blood vessels, but each of these drugs does so in a slightly different way. Avastin works by binding to vascular endothelial growth factor (VEGF), which is a signaling molecule that leads normal endothelial cells—the cells that line the interior of blood vessels—to grow new blood vessels. Avastin blocks the VEGF receptors and stops the growth of the tumor's blood supply.[11] Since it approved Avastin in 2004, the FDA has approved other drugs of this type, including sorafenib, sunitinib, pazopanib, and everolimus. These other angiogenesis inhibitors bind to receptors on the surface of endothelial cells or to other proteins that provide growth signals, in order to block signals that lead to the creation of new blood cells to feed the tumor.[12]

Drugs of this type can slow the growth of the tumor, and in some cases, these therapies may shrink the tumor. For some cancers, there is evidence that these drugs extend patients' lives. At the same time, these drugs can also have serious side effects. These can include bleeding, clots in the arteries leading to stroke or heart attack, and protein in the urine, because angiogenesis is a process that is also necessary for many normal functions.[13] Even though the risks are considerable, the potential of Avastin and other antiangiogenesis drugs to prolong the lives of women living with metastatic breast cancer and the desire of Genentech to expand the market for its drug led the push to make this drug available for this population as soon as possible. To understand the regulatory framework that led to the accelerated approval of Avastin, we start with a description of the U.S. drug approval process and the development of the FDA's expedited approval programs.

Drug Regulation in the United States: From Caveat Emptor to Accelerated Approval

Until the early 20th century, the United States relied on a market-based approach and allowed individual patients to decide what to buy, often based on suggestions from a physician. The principle of caveat emptor, "let the buyer beware," shaped the government's approach to drugs and devices. Under this system, many of the so-called medicines sold by pharmacists and small-business owners who promoted their products in almanacs, magazines, and medicine shows had little if any evidence to support their clinical effectiveness. The ingredients in many of the products sold included opium, cocaine, and alcohol. When people were harmed by these products, the remedy was the tort system.

Progressive Era Reforms

The first shift away from the market-oriented approach to food and drugs occurred during the Progressive Era of the early 20th century, when muckraking journalists and novelists exposed troubling industry practices that threatened the health and well-being of workers and the public. One of the most well-known exposés was Upton Sinclair's novel *The Jungle*, which documented the unsanitary practices of the meat-packing industry. Journalist Samuel Hopkins Adams, writing for *Collier's Weekly*, had a similar impact on the pharmaceutical industry. In an eleven-article series titled "The Great American Fraud," he criticized the patent medicine industry for marketing products that failed to offer effective therapies and often put the public's health at risk by including alcohol, opioids, and other dangerous ingredients in their products.[14] The Proprietary Association, which represented the manufacturers of patent medicine, lobbied to block the inclusion of these drugs in the proposed bill to regulate foods, but the AMA lobbied in favor of regulating drugs because they were often marketed as potential substitutes for physician services.[15] Public reaction to the muckraking reports, coupled with the support of organized medicine and President Theodore Roosevelt, led Congress to adopt the Pure Food and Drug Act of 1906. The law banned foreign and interstate traffic in adulterated or mislabeled food and drug products, and it required manufacturers to place the active ingredient of a drug on the label and to make sure that drugs did not fall below purity standards.[16] Even after the adoption of the law, the FDA did not have the authority to require preapproval of drugs before they were sold on the market. Instead, the agency only took action after it detected violations of the law.

The Food, Drug, and Cosmetic Act of 1938

In 1938 the U.S. government adopted a more aggressive approach to food and drug regulation when Congress adopted the FDCA. Momentum for stricter regulation of pharmaceutical products began to grow during the 1930s due to increasing concern about products that harmed or killed consumers. The issue of drug regulation was not high on President Franklin Roosevelt's policy agenda, but in 1933, Senator Royal S. Copeland (D-NY) introduced the "Tugwell Bill." The bill was named after Assistant Secretary of Agriculture Rexford G. Tugwell, who was alarmed by popular accounts of harmful food and drug products and initiated the effort to revise the 1906 law.[17] The proposal for a new act was met with fierce resistance from both the food and drug industries. The FDA countered this opposition by creating a public exhibit documenting an array of products that had harmed individuals.[18] Industry opposition and a lack of strong support from the president helped to stall the bill in Congress. As with more contemporary drug industry opposition to regulations that interfere with patient and physician autonomy, the drug industry argued that the proposed bill would "deprive the American people of their right to 'self-medication.'"[19] In 1937, however, a "focusing event" helped to improve the proposal's fortunes. In that year, a drug known as "Elixir Sulfanilamide," sold by the Massengill Company (sulfanilamide with diethylene glycol, a solvent) poisoned 100 people.[20] This tragedy was used by the bill's proponents to secure the votes necessary for passage.

The 1938 Act, which was signed into law by President Roosevelt on June 25, required companies to submit a new drug application (NDA), which provided premarket notification of the safety of a drug before it could be marketed. The FDA was required to render a decision in 60 days. If the FDA did not act to reject the drug within this time frame, it could be marketed. The agency could reject a drug within this window if the manufacturer neglected to submit evidence that it had failed to conduct adequate safety tests, if the results of those tests suggested that the drug was unsafe, or if there was evidence that the manufacturer could not preserve the "identity, strength, quality and purity" of the product.[21] The act also required that drug manufacturers comply with investigational new drug (IND) regulations before they could test a compound on humans.[22] The law authorized the secretary of the U.S. Department of Agriculture to exempt new drugs used for experimental purposes by qualified experts. (In 1940 the FDA was transferred to the Federal Security Agency, which became the Department of Health, Education, and Welfare in 1953 and the Department of Health and Human Services in 1979.) The law did not, however, require manufacturers to test whether a new compound was therapeutically effective.

The 1962 Kefauver-Harris Drug Amendments

In 1962, President Kennedy signed into law Kefauver-Harris Drug Amendments to the Food, Drug and Cosmetic Act, which significantly strengthened the ability of the FDA to regulate the safety of drugs.[23] As with the 1938 Act, the changes were driven by the response to tragedy. The amendments were introduced into Congress in response to the use of Thalidomide in Europe in the early 1960s. Thalidomide was used to treat pregnancy-related illnesses for women but resulted in birth defects in thousands of babies. The FDA had not allowed Thalidomide to be marketed in the United States, but the public reaction to this tragedy still generated calls for stricter drug regulations. The 1962 amendments replaced the 1938 system of premarket notification with a requirement that companies must receive premarket approval from the FDA before a drug could be sold. In addition, the 1962 amendments introduced a requirement that manufacturers demonstrate effectiveness, usually by conducting two controlled clinical trials. The amendments also required companies to adhere to stricter manufacturing practices and to conduct postmarketing surveillance by monitoring safety reports after the drugs reached the market.

To implement the 1962 amendments, the FDA promulgated a new standard of research required to support an NDA. First, in order to receive an IND to begin human testing, a manufacturer must provide the FDA with a plan for human research and a report with any known data on the compound, including human experiences with the drug and animal toxicology studies. Once the IND is granted, a company is required to go through three phases of clinical investigation. Phase I involves a study on a small number of volunteers and is designed to test for appropriate dosages, toxicity, and provide initial information about effectiveness. Phase II is a controlled study of a few hundred patients to evaluate the effectiveness of the drug and determine side effects. Phase III trials are large RCTs designed to determine therapeutic effectiveness. The FDA usually requires two Phase III trials before it will approve an NDA, though some drugs have been approved under an accelerated approval pathway after completion of Phase II trials.[24]

The process and standards put in place by the 1962 amendments helped to solidify the FDA's reputation as a world leader in drug regulation, frequently touted as a gold standard around the world. The discovery of acquired immune deficiency syndrome (AIDS) in the early 1980s, however, raised questions about whether FDA standards were too strict and the process of drug approval too slow to respond adequately to this crisis. Efforts by physicians and AIDS advocacy groups helped to bring about substantial changes that, over time, led to expedited drug development and approval programs for serious conditions.

In the early 1980s, health officials began to notice a new disease in young, white, gay men, particularly in Los Angeles, New York City, and San Francisco. Because the most obvious symptom of this new disease was purple skin tumors associated with Kaposi's sarcoma, many referred to the disease as "gay cancer." No one understood the cause of the disease, and its spread caused alarm in the gay community.

Activists around the country worked with remarkable speed and energy to organize to provide support and treatment to those who became sick—and to push for government action to confront the crisis. New York writer Larry Kramer organized a meeting at his apartment to raise money for research, which led to the establishment of the Gay Men's Health Crisis Center in 1982. In 1983, the AIDS Medical Foundation (AMF) was established to raise money for research, and it awarded its first research grants in 1984. AMF also worked to disseminate information about the disease to public officials and the general public. In September 1985, AMF merged with the National AIDS Research Foundation, which was established in California in 1985, to form the American Foundation for AIDS Research, the largest organization dedicated to AIDS research and policy.[25]

AIDS activists played an important role in increasing public awareness and raising money for research, but their major policy accomplishments focused on changes in policies that govern the research, testing, evaluation, and dissemination of new medical treatments. AIDS activism "resulted in the *multiplication of the successful pathways* to the establishment of credibility and *diversification of the personnel* beyond the highly credentialed."[26] By immersing themselves in the technical details and language of the process, AIDS activists revolutionized the procedures for testing and licensing of new drugs.[27] Their extensive knowledge of the disease gave HIV/AIDS activists credibility with scientists and policymakers and enhanced the effectiveness of their lobbying efforts.[28]

Expedited Approval and Expanded Access

In response to the AIDS crisis, the FDA developed multiple pathways for faster approval of specialty drugs, particularly for life-threatening conditions.[29] By 1983 Congress had already passed the Orphan Drug Act, which was intended to encourage drug companies to develop treatments for rare diseases. Eventually, this law became linked with the development of treatments for AIDS patients. Notably, zidovudine and zalcitabine both received orphan drug status for the treatment of what was then called AIDS-related complex—but the original push for this legislation preceded the AIDS crisis.[30]

A more direct response to the AIDS crisis took place in 1988 when the FDA created a "fast track" designation that allows early approval of drugs for life-threatening illness or debilitating disease on the basis of Phase II clinical trial results indicating some evidence for clinical effectiveness.[31] In 1992 the FDA also formalized its priority review designation, a version of which had been in place since 1975, to guarantee a "review of new drug applications within six months of submission for drugs seeming to offer a therapeutic advance over available therapy."[32] Accelerated approval, authorized by Congress in 1992, was used to secure FDA approval for the use of Avastin to treat advanced breast cancer. Accelerated approval allows the agency to approve a drug to treat serious or life-threatening illnesses based on early clinical trial results using "surrogate" end points, like reductions in tumor size or improvements in progression-free survival, that are likely to predict patient benefit. It is important to note that surrogate end points are frequently used by the FDA to make decisions about drugs that do not involve accelerated approval. That is because some surrogates are very well established as reliable markers for clinical benefit. In the case of accelerated approval, the FDA relaxes that standard and will consider the use of surrogate end points (like progression-free survival) that are not yet established in the literature "but are 'reasonably likely' to predict improved clinical outcomes." Unfortunately, the "reasonably likely" standard has never been defined by the FDA.[33]

While the lack of clarity about the "reasonable and likely" standard provides the agency with flexibility, it means there is often debate about whether a surrogate end point is sufficient. It also places great importance on the need for conducting postapproval trials "in a timely and rigorous manner."[34] As FDA officials explained during the hearing to debate the 2011 Avastin decision, "this kind of accelerated approval is subject to a requirement that the applicant must perform additional, well controlled clinical investigations to verify and describe the expected clinical benefit."[35] If subsequent evidence does not support the continued use of the drug that was approved conditionally under the accelerated pathway, the FDA is supposed to withdraw approval. Frequently, at least two factors can interfere with this process. First, drug companies often do not complete postapproval trials in a timely manner—sometimes taking several years, and in some cases, more than a decade to do so. Second, the decision can be politically difficult because the manufacturer, along with physicians and patients who are using the approved drug, have a strong stake in maintaining approval and are often supported by members of Congress who oppose actions by the government to reduce access to new drugs—regardless of the strength of evidence behind them.

In 2012 Congress codified the FDA's accelerated approval pathway and added another pathway for faster approval of so-called "breakthrough" therapies.[36] According to the 2012 Food and Drug Administration Safety and Innovation Act, a breakthrough therapy is one that is

> intended alone or in combination with one or more other drugs to treat a serious or life threatening disease or condition and preliminary clinical evidence indicates that the drug may demonstrate substantial improvement over existing therapies on one or more clinically significant endpoints, such as substantial treatment effects observed early in clinical development.[37]

The various pathways described above were supposed to be used infrequently in cases for which there was promising initial evidence that a drug could offer improved outcomes for patients suffering from life-threatening illnesses.[38] Research suggests that, rather than being rare events, approval through these pathways has become common and now represents about a quarter of all drug approvals. According to a 2015 General Accountability Office (GAO) report, drug companies submitted 772 requests for some form of fast-track designation between 2007 and 2015, two-thirds of which were approved by the FDA.[39] Between 2012, when the process was established, and 2015, companies submitted 225 requests for breakthrough therapy designation. The FDA approved just under half of these requests.

Not only are the mechanisms for expediting the drug development and approval process used with much greater frequency than originally imagined by Congress or the FDA, there are concerns that the postapproval studies that allow the agency to assess the appropriateness of its original accelerated approval decision are often not completed in a timely fashion. The GAO concluded that "the FDA lacks reliable, readily accessible data on tracked safety issues and postmarket studies needed to meet certain postmarket safety reporting responsibilities and to conduct systematic oversight."[40] The case of Avastin illustrates why conducting such studies is so important when drugs are approved on the basis of limited evidence.

Conditional Approval to Use Avastin for Treating Advanced Breast Cancer

In 2006 the FDA approved the use of Avastin as a first-line treatment for advanced nonsquamous non-small-cell lung cancer in combination with carboplatin and paclitaxel.[41] The 2006 approval was based on trials that showed that Avastin was associated with improvements in overall survival among these patients, although other trials in Europe did not replicate this finding and were only able to demonstrate an improvement in progression-free survival.[42] In 2008 the drug received accelerated approval by the FDA to treat metastatic breast cancer,[43] but the agency revoked its approval for this indication in 2011. The basis for the 2008 decision to receive accelerated approval for the use of Avastin for advanced breast cancer were findings from the E2100 trial, published in the *New England Journal of Medicine (NEJM)* in 2007. This trial indicated that Avastin, used in combination with paclitaxel, was able to increase progression-free survival among women in the trial from 5.8 to 11.3 months, compared with women who used paclitaxel alone, with modest increases in toxicity among most women.[44] A second trial, AVF2119g, did not find improvements in progression-free or overall survival.[45] The drug's producer, Genentech, distributed copies of the *NEJM* article widely to encourage the use of Avastin for breast cancer patients among physicians. By the time the drug received approval from the FDA for its use as a breast cancer treatment, about 9,000 breast cancer patients in the United States had received an off-label prescription of Avastin.[46]

The FDA's Oncologic Drugs Advisory Committee (ODAC), which included seven experts in the field of oncology or statistics and two consumer representatives, held a meeting to consider accelerated approval for Avastin in combination with paclitaxel, as a first-line treatment for advanced breast cancer, on December 5, 2007.[47] Members of the ODAC questioned the strength of the evidence in favor of using Avastin for the treatment of advanced breast cancer and voted five to four against approval. Along with concerns about the design of the E2100 trials, members of the committee questioned whether the improvements in progression-free survival were sufficient, because the hazard ratios presented suggested that adding Avastin to paclitaxel was unlikely to lead to an improvement in overall survival. In their clinical review of the evidence to ODAC, Drs. Lee Pai-Scherf and Hong Lu of the FDA concluded that the E2100 trial was able to establish an increase in progression-free survival, but the evidence for the magnitude of this effect (5.5-month improvement in progression-free survival) was not reliable because 10 percent of the scans were missing, 34 percent of patients were not followed to the end of the study, and the trial investigators and independent radiologists did not agree about the trial's findings with regard to the radiologic disease progression.[48] Furthermore, they concluded that the E2100 trial had an incomplete assessment of the drug's toxicity profile for breast cancer patients because information about grade 1 and 2 toxicity were not collected and laboratory data were not collected. In addition, the E2100 trial found a 20.2 percent increase in grade 3–5 toxicity, which represents life-threatening events, and a small increase in treatment-related deaths among patients in the bevacizumab plus paclitaxel arm.[49]

Despite the ODAC vote, the FDA granted accelerated approval for the breast cancer indication in 2008, which meant that subsequent data from additional clinical trials must be presented to the FDA in order to confirm the drug's clinical benefit.[50] The FDA required Genentech to submit data from two ongoing trials (AVADO and RIBBON1) to verify the treatment effect on progression-free survival found in the E2100 trial and to provide additional information on the effects on overall survival.

Reversing Course

On November 16, 2009, just over one year after the initial FDA decision, Genentech submitted the results of the AVADO and RIBBON1 trials to the FDA's Center for Drug Evaluation and Research (CDER) in compliance with the requirements of accelerated approval of Avastin's breast cancer indication.[51] Eight months later, on July 2, 2010, the ODAC met to review the results from the Avastin to docetaxel (AVADO trial) and the taxane/anthracycline-based chemotherapy to capecitabine (RIBBON1 trial). Both trials provided further evidence of gains in progression-free survival, but the magnitude of the effect was smaller than the one documented by the E2100 trial. As with the two previous trials, neither the AVADO nor RIBBON1 trials demonstrated an improvement in overall survival, nor did they provide evidence of improvements in patient-reported outcomes, like disease-related symptoms or health-related quality of life. In addition, there was an overall increase in serious, life-threatening adverse events related to Avastin. These included increases in hypertension, bleeding/hemorrhage, wound-healing complications, perforation and fistula/abscess formation, arterial thromboembolic events (stroke, myocardial infarction), venous embolic events, febrile neutropenia, left ventricular dysfunction, and reversible posterior leukoencephalopathy.[52]

On the basis of these new findings from the AVADO and RIBBON1 trials, coupled with the concerns that were raised in 2008 on the basis of the E2100 and AVF2119g trials, ODAC voted twelve to one to recommend withdrawing the FDA's accelerated approval of the first-line breast cancer indication for Avastin. On the basis of the ODAC recommendation, CDER proposed that the FDA withdraw marketing approval for Avastin to treat metastatic breast cancer, specifically for use in combination with paclitaxel for the treatment of patients who have not had chemotherapy for metastatic HER2 negative breast cancer. The FDA announced, in December 2010 that it would start the process of withdrawing its approval for Avastin's breast cancer indication. Genentech, which stood to lose $1 billion in sales as a result of the decision, filed an opposition petition and requested an administrative hearing.[53]

June 2011 FDA Hearing

On June 28 and 29, 2011, the FDA conducted a hearing on the CDER's proposal.[54] During the first two hours of the hearing, 14 advocacy organizations, 17 individual women who were living with breast cancer, and four individual oncologists offered testimony to the FDA about the proposal to withdraw market approval for Avastin for the breast cancer indication. The National Breast Cancer Coalition (NBBC), which had raised concerns about the 2008 decision to approve the indication for Avastin, expressed strong support for CDER's recommendation. All of the other organizations and individuals who testified at the hearing voiced opposition to the recommendation. In addition, the FDA continued to allow the public to submit comments about the proposal for withdrawing market approval until July 28, 2011.[55] The agency received around 450 comments, most of which were from patients who opposed the proposed action.[56]

Accusations of FDA Bias

Abigail Alliance for Better Access to Developmental Drugs testified in opposition to the proposed withdrawal of FDA approval for the breast cancer indication. The position of Abigail Alliance was not surprising because advocating for access to unapproved drugs—and against efforts by the FDA to limit access to drugs—is the reason for the organization's existence. Abigail Alliance was formed in 2001 by the father of a 19-year-old woman, Abigail Burroughs, who was denied access under the FDA's "compassionate use exception" rules to an unapproved drug to treat her terminal head and neck cancer. In 2003 the Abigail Alliance sued the FDA, arguing that the agency had violated the 14th Amendment of the U.S. Constitution by denying access to unapproved drugs. In 2006 the U.S. Court of Appeals for the District of Columbia heard *Abigail Alliance for Better Access to Developmental Drugs v. Von Eschenbach*, and a three-judge panel ruled in favor of Abigail Alliance. A year later, however, the FDA appealed the decision, and an en banc review overturned the appeals court's decision and found that there is no constitutional right to access to experimental therapies.[57]

At the 2011 FDA hearing, the Abigail Alliance asserted that Avastin was effective, but they did not offer any evidence in support of this assertion. Instead, their representative focused on what they viewed as FDA bias. The Abigail Alliance representative argued that Richard Pazdur, MD, the director of the FDA's Oncology Center of Excellence, had selected voting members of the ODAC who would tip the balance in favor of the committee recommending that the FDA withdraw Avastin's market approval for the breast cancer indication.[58]

The accusation by the Abigail Alliance was ironic because Dr. Pazdur has been criticized by some for being too enthusiastic about new cancer drugs. In 2013, referring to new cancer drugs in the pipeline, Dr. Pazdur argued that the FDA did not "have a lot of questions on [these] drugs because they're slam dunks. It's not *if* we're going to approve them. It's how fast we're going to approve them."[59] Critics contend that the FDA routinely approves new cancer drugs based on trials that are methodologically weak and enjoy "an easy ride from regulators for drugs that usually offer few significant benefits for patients."[60] Nevertheless, the proposal to withdraw market approval for Avastin generated anger among those who still did not believe the FDA was doing enough to speed access to drugs.

Progression-Free vs. Overall Survival

All four oncologists who testified opposed the FDA proposal to withdraw approval. They argued that a decision to withdraw approval for Avastin for their breast cancer patients would be, in the words of one, "devastating." One physician raised the issue of progression-free survival as an end point. He questioned the standards of the FDA and wondered why evidence of progression-free survival was insufficient for continued approval. His argument was, in part, a call for consistency. He argued that the FDA had "approved other drugs with only progression-free survival without overall survival. You approved Ixempra. You approved Tykerb. Why can't you leave Avastin on the market?"[61] The concern about relying on overall survival was also articulated by a number of the advocacy groups who testified, including groups representing patients with other forms of cancer for whom this is also a crucial issue. For example, the Ovarian Cancer National Alliance, a patient advocacy group (which had received funding from Genentech), argued that "progression-free survival or PFS is often the most objective and, hence, most valid endpoint in a clinical trial."[62]

This statement reflects the view, shared by many in the pharmaceutical industry and patient advocacy communities, that progression-free survival, because it is easier to measure, is a more valid and reliable end point. Those who adopt this perspective also argue that trial designs that are frequently used in cancer trials make it difficult to establish changes in overall survival. In particular, there is concern that overall survival is a problematic end point in trials, like those used to investigate Avastin that use crossover designs. In such trials, patients are permitted to "cross over" to the alternate arm of the trial after disease progression. The argument is that these trials measure the effects of a treatment sequence, not just the effect of the new treatment. This design makes it difficult to establish the effect of the new treatment's improved overall survival—and this is why it is an unfair standard.[63]

In contrast, the NBCC, which had been opposed to the original approval of the use of Avastin for metastatic breast cancer, voiced strong support for the FDA proposal to withdraw approval for the indication. In doing so, it reiterated the case for looking at overall survival. At the FDA hearing, Christine Brunswick, who was the vice president of the NBCC and also living with metastatic breast cancer, testified that

> Avastin has been shown to be unsafe and ineffective for breast cancer patients. The FDA's decision on Avastin must be based on scientific evidence from well-done trials and cannot be based on any one individual story, no matter how compelling. This decision cannot be driven by anecdotes. It must be driven by science. This decision must be made for the greater good and on a public health basis. The addition of Avastin failed to demonstrate a significant improvement in overall survival. This may not be what many of us wanted to hear, but we must accept and act on evidence or we will never make the needed progress we so desperately want.[64]

Ms. Brunswick's contrast between anecdotes and science hints at the divisions about what counts as evidence that animate the Avastin story and the other cases in this book. Furthermore, the doubts articulated by Ms. Brunswick on behalf of NBCC about the validity of progression-free survival as a valid end point for evaluating Avastin were shared by FDA officials. The dispute between individuals and groups who testified in favor of continuing to rely on progression-free survival and those who argued that this was insufficient for longer-term approval is driven in part by a lack of evidence about how well progression-free survival is measured, but also about the relationship between progression-free and overall survival. One meta-analysis of the relevant literature found that there have been only three individual-patient-level randomized trials with evidence about the relationship between surrogate and final end points for metastatic cancer—and only one for breast cancer. These trials found "modest correlations" between these two end points, leaving plenty of room for skepticism on both sides of the debate.[65] As one scholar explained, finding that a drug has an effect on a surrogate measure establishes that there is biological activity, but "may not provide reliable evidence about effects of the intervention on clinical efficacy measures."[66] It is possible that a disease independently affects the surrogate end point and the clinical end point. If this is the case, a change in the surrogate end point may have no implications for whether the drug will affect the clinical end point. Another possibility is that the surrogate is a marker for one causal pathway of disease but not other pathways. Finally, the drug could have a positive impact on a surrogate end point that is causally related to the clinical end point but also has other effects that lead to other problems and make it more likely that people experience poor clinical outcomes.[67] In all of these scenarios, it may be possible to alter the surrogate end point but not improve the health of the patient.

But the disagreement goes beyond a lack of evidence or the complexity of interpreting evidence. While there is dispute about whether it is realistic to find differences in overall survival in trials for drugs designed to investigate solid tumors, there is also a disagreement about the value of progression-free survival to patients. If we had broadly accepted evidence that a drug delayed the progression of a metastatic disease but did not result in overall survival, some would argue that the drug is still valuable because delayed progression is a worthy goal. Several of the patients who testified before the FDA in 2011 articulated this perspective, and it is a view that is also accepted by some oncologists. Others, however, argue that this does not represent a benefit to patients and merely lowers "the bar to declare active some of our much-heralded new molecular targeted therapies."[68] As such, the debate over end points not only involves technical disagreements about how to measure these outcomes, how to validate the measures, and how to design trials in ways that make it more likely that the outcomes will be reliable; they involve debates about the goals of treatment. These debates involve nonscientific questions that cannot be resolved by evidence alone.

Possibility of Super Responders

The individual patients who testified at the hearing had all used Avastin and attributed positive outcomes to the drug. They pleaded with the FDA officials not to withdraw approval for a treatment that, from their perspective, had allowed them to continue living. Many of the women referred to themselves as "super responders." This term is invoked frequently in the literature on pharmaceuticals, particularly in connection with cancer drugs. The idea is that, even though a drug may appear to be ineffective for most of the patients who use it, there is a small subset of people (called "super" or "exceptional" responders) for whom the drug is highly effective. Much of the enthusiasm about so-called "precision medicine" is the idea that physicians will be able to use the results of genetic tests to identify drugs that will work particularly well for a specific patient. By targeting drugs to patients on the basis of particular gene mutations, the hope is that precision medicine will make it easier to find and treat so-called super responders. Despite the excitement around precision medicine, there is little evidence to date that genetic tests are able to generate results of this sort for most cancer patients.[69] Similarly, although there is a growing literature with reports of super responders, evidence of underlying biological explanations for these results are, at best, incomplete.[70] In its review of the trial results for Avastin, the

FDA specifically looked for evidence of possible super responders and concluded that no such evidence existed. The agency contended that the data "had not shown even a small subset of women receiving Avastin living substantially longer than those in the control group, raising doubts about whether there are 'super responders' who derive great benefit from the drug."[71] Nevertheless, there was strong belief among many of the women who testified, and many others who offered written comments to the FDA through the *Federal Register*, that their experiences supported the existence of super responders.

A woman with recurrent metastatic cancer who had been on Avastin for three years claimed, "I am a super responder. I have virtually no side effects. I have a runny nose, and the protein in my urine rises about twice a year. I drink more water, and it drops. [My physician] continues to monitor my cancer and feels like Avastin is the proper treatment for me. My recent bone and body scan show that I remain to be in remission almost three years later because of Avastin."[72] The husband of a woman being treated with Avastin accused the FDA of behaving irresponsibly, called for a congressional investigation of the agency, and argued that its understanding of evidence was flawed. He focused specifically on the issue of disaggregation. "Despite strong empirical and observed evidence, the FDA contemptuously ignores these women, dismissively calling them 'anecdotal evidence' . . . [t]he FDA unscientifically only considers medians from its trials. However, the FDA approach misleadingly omits the details behind the medians."[73]

A representative from an advocacy group Facing Our Risk of Cancer Empowered also invoked the idea of super responders and suggested that women with the BRCA gene might be one of the groups who benefitted from Avastin more than others. She argued that "research shows that certain women with metastatic breast cancer benefit from the drug. Although we do not yet know who benefits most, we know that BRCA-associated cancers respond to certain treatments differently than sporadic cancers, and there is anecdotal evidence to suggest that BRCA mutation patients may be among those that respond well."[74]

A woman with metastatic breast cancer since 2007 who participated in one of the Avastin trials attributed her continued survival to the drug. She argued that, regardless of the aggregate results, she and some other women responded well to the drug. Another woman with metastatic breast cancer diagnosed in 2009 gave a detailed account of her cancer experience and questioned why studies focused on average results should be used to discount her experience. As she put it:

At the time of my diagnosis, I had 14 tumors in my liver, over 30 in my lungs, and two in my spine. I was in excruciating around-the-clock pain. After three months of Avastin and Abraxane, the tumors in my body had decreased in size by nearly 50 percent, the hypermetabolic activity was greatly reduced, and my pain was nearly eliminated. By June of last year, all my tumors were quiet and many had resolved completely. I tolerated Avastin extremely well with very minimal side effects. I understand and appreciate that academic research typically and appropriately discounts anecdotal evidence. But isn't the scientific evidence merely a collection of individual anecdotes? . . . In spite of disappointing survival benefit, Avastin has been shown to improve progression-free disease, which from a patient's perspective cannot be understated.[75]

Several additional women living with metastatic cancer presented their cases and told comparable stories. One referred to Avastin as her "miracle drug" and claimed that Avastin had led to clean PET scans and a normal life for three years. Each of these stories is deeply moving and helps to explain why some oppose the FDA's decision to withdraw approval for this indication. They do not, however, answer the question of how much weight, if any, should be placed on these individual stories in light of the evidence from multiple, randomized clinical trials.

Patient and Physician Autonomy

A third theme that emerged from the hearing was the idea of patient and physician autonomy. This was related to the claims about super responders in the sense that these arguments also focused on the importance of individual-level results, but they added to this an argument about the extent to which individuals should be allowed to make their own decisions about how to weigh benefits and harms. Several women who testified mentioned that they had signed a consent form when they agreed to take the drug and that they were well aware of the potential harms associated with it. As one woman put it, "Like all other treatments I've received over the years, I signed an informed consent prior to receiving Avastin. I understood the risks and potential benefits."[76] Another woman with triple negative metastatic breast cancer pointed out that she was a nurse and aware of the risks associated with Avastin and other treatment options. A third woman not only invoked the fact that she had signed an informed consent document but emphasized the degree to which she made the decision to use the drug in consultation with her physicians. She said, "I have given my informed consent to be treated with Avastin. I do sometimes worry about the side effects and the long-term damages that can be done, but the bottom line is my cardiologist assists in my medical management along with my oncologist by understanding, monitoring and treating for the drug's effects. My oncologist and I are both fairly certain I wouldn't be here right now if it weren't for Avastin. I would be dead."[77] The view that patients and physicians should be empowered to make decisions about how to balance benefits and harms was repeated throughout the hearing.

Along with the representative from NBCC, one other member of the public attempted to counter the patient and physician autonomy narrative. Helen Schiff—who represented SHARE leaders, a group of cancer survivors and graduates from NBCC's advocacy training program—suggested that the overwhelming number of testimonies from people who opposed the FDA decision was not representative. Although she expressed support for "allow[ing] women already responding to Avastin-containing regimes to stay on them," she asked the committee to remember that most women who were harmed by Avastin could not come forward to testify.

> While I have a few seconds, just in my own name I would like to say that for every woman here testifying, there are other women who we know—a member of our group who bled out of every orifice of her body, Jimke Vassu; another woman, Sandra—I can't remember her last name—in Florida who had a brain hemorrhage. So those people don't come to testify. I just want you to remember that they exist, too.[78]

At the end of the hearing, the ODAC unanimously recommended that the FDA withdraw market approval of Avastin for the breast cancer indication, and about five months after the ODAC vote, FDA commissioner Margaret Hamburg announced that the agency would do so. Hamburg's decision was met with an outcry from many patients and their advocates, as well as several members of Congress. Although Medicare initially continued to pay for the off-label use of Avastin among breast cancer patients, and several large health insurance companies decided to do the same, there was no guarantee they would continue to do so. In response to Hamburg's decision, Representative Sue Myrick (R-NC) expressed concern that breast cancer patients who wanted to continue their treatment with the drug off label would be unable to do so. She said, "when a drug can help save patients' lives, they should be able to do that affordably. Insurers now could cut off coverage, and not pay for the drug."[79]

Conclusions: Avastin and the Push for Faster Approval

The case of Avastin highlights the dangers of the FDA's expedited drug development and approval programs—particularly the accelerated approval pathway—because these programs may allow the use of drugs for which there is inadequate evidence of benefit and significant risk of harm. At the same time, the case also provides evidence that the FDA was willing to act on updated information and make the unpopular decision to revoke approval based on postapproval studies. Daniel Carpenter, one of the leading experts on the FDA, argues that the Avastin decision reflects a willingness of the agency to assert its independence, even though it faced great pressure from Congress, the drug's sponsor, and a host of advocacy groups to retain market approval for the drug. Despite this, he also argues that the amount of time the agency took to finally reach a decision in this case, with long delays between the submission of new trial data and the final decision to withdraw approval, undermines confidence in the agency. As he put it, "This kind of delay looks bad, not least because the scientific opinion has been clarified, making any lag seem to be caused by the worst form of politics. Once the advisory committee has voted on an issue, the commissioner should have no more than a month to make a decision."[80]

An even bigger concern raised by the Avastin case is the implications of poor industry compliance with confirmatory studies. The use of existing accelerated approvals and the pressure to move even faster place great importance on the existence of timely, reliable postmarket confirmatory studies. In the case of Avastin, the additional trials were completed relatively soon after the initial decision, but often that is not the case. Unless the FDA is willing to enforce the "mandatory" completion of such studies, it will not be possible for the agency, members of Congress, or members of the public at large to evaluate whether accelerated approvals helped secure fast access to an effective drug—or exposed the public to a harmful drug approved on the basis of limited evidence.

The Path to the Clinic for Stem Cell and Other Regenerative Medicine Interventions

Stem cell interventions are part of a suite of interventions from the medical field—and the commercial biotechnology product sector—known as regenerative medicine. Developing interventions in regenerative medicine involves the "process of replenishing or restoring human cells, tissues, or organs to restore or reestablish normal function."[1] These interventions have their roots in decades of transplantation research involving humans and nonhuman animals.[2] According to the Alliance for Regenerative Medicine, a membership organization composed of pharmaceutical and biotechnology companies, investors, university-based and nonprofit research institutions, patient advocacy groups, and researchers, by the end of 2016, more than 700 companies, including divisions of multinational corporations and small biotech firms, focused solely on regenerative medicine and related advanced therapies.[3]

The human body contains nearly 200 different types of cells that perform different functions. Stem cells hold great therapeutic promise because as unspecialized cells, they can renew themselves and be induced under certain physiologic or experimental conditions to become tissue- or organ-specific cells with special functions. "Embryonic stem cells" are derived from early human embryos, whereas "adult stem cells" are found in many tissues in the human body. Adult stem cells include but are not limited to hematopoietic stem cells (derived from bone marrow and umbilical cord blood), neural stem cells found in the brain, and mesenchymal stem cells that have been isolated from adipose tissue (body fat), placenta, bone marrow, and blood.

An autologous stem cell intervention involves collecting stem cells from a patient, processing them in various ways, and then infusing the processed cells into the same patient. An allogeneic intervention involves infusing into patients cultured stem cells that were derived from donors.[4]

By the late 1990s, the therapeutic breakthroughs in human organ transplantation and in bone marrow transplantation for some types of blood diseases and breast cancers raised expectations that therapeutic treatments using stem cells were just around the corner. Nonetheless, the National Research Council and Institute of Medicine pointed out in their 2002 report, *Stem Cells and the Future of Regenerative Medicine*, that scientists still had much to learn about the therapeutic potential of human stem cells.[5] The limited evidence of the safety and effectiveness of stem cell interventions other than hematopoietic stem cell transplants did not, however, keep some physicians and clinics from offering patients such interventions.

In late 2008, the journal *Cell Stem Cell* published the findings of a study that examined the Web sites of 19 clinics outside the United States to determine how the clinics were advertising stem cell interventions for which there was little or no evidence of safety and effectiveness from clinical trials. The study found that 47 percent of the clinics offered autologous adult stem cell interventions, 32 percent offered interventions using fetal stem cells, 21 percent offered interventions from cord blood, with the others offering embryonic stem cell interventions or allogeneic adult stem cell interventions. The stem cells for the interventions were derived primarily from bone marrow (37 percent), with 26 percent coming from the blood or marrow donors, and 26 percent from peripheral blood. Stem cells were also derived from fetuses, body fat, "unspecified," and "other." Neurologic conditions, cardiovascular disease, multiple sclerosis, stroke, Parkinson's disease, spinal cord injury, and Alzheimer's disease were the conditions most often cited on the Web sites as those the stem cell interventions were designed to treat. A few clinics also said they offered stem cell interventions to treat several conditions diagnosed in children, such as cerebral palsy, autism, and Duchenne muscular dystrophy.[6]

No clinics in the United States were included in the study, and little was known at the time of publication how many companies in the United States were developing and marketing stem cell interventions or how many physicians were offering these interventions to their patients. But the spotlight shifted to the United States when the FDA investigated a Colorado company that was marketing a stem cell intervention for which it had not obtained premarket approval from the agency. As for treatments involving traditional medical drugs, patients should receive stem cell interventions only if they are safe and effective. Yet because stem cell interventions are different from traditional medical drugs and may involve surgical and other procedures, whether and how the FDA should regulate these interventions—and what evidentiary standards for showing the interventions are safe and effective—are questions at the center of a longstanding dispute that took a new turn when Congress passed the 21st Century Cures Act in 2016.

FDA Regulation of Cellular Products

The FDA regulates the development, distribution, and market entry of drugs under the FDCA and regulates biological products under the Public Health Service (PHS) Act. The FDCA defines a drug as an article "intended for use in the diagnosis, cure, mitigation, treatment, or prevention of disease" or "intended to affect the structure or any function of the body of man or other animals."[7] A biological product under the PHS Act is defined as a "virus, therapeutic serum, toxin, antitoxin, vaccine, blood, blood component or derivative, allergenic product, protein (except any chemically synthesized polypeptide), or analogous product . . . applicable to the prevention, treatment, or cure of a disease or condition of human beings."[8]

With advances in scientific research in the 1990s, there was growing recognition of the therapeutic potential of human cells, tissues, and cellular and tissue-based products (HCT/Ps). For the FDA and agencies in other countries that regulated the market entry of medical products, an important question was whether and how to regulate market entry for interventions using these types of human biological materials.

The 2001 Rule

The FDA issued a final rule in 2001 to regulate different types of HCT/Ps that consisted of human cells or tissues "intended for implantation, transplantation, infusion or transfer into human recipients."[9] The agency adopted a risk-based regulatory approach to increase the safety of HCT/Ps, foster public confidence in their safety, and encourage scientific innovation. Under the 2001 rule, HCT/Ps are regulated as a drug, device, and/or biological product if they are not intended for homologous use only and do not meet criteria about how and the extent to which cells and structural and nonstructural tissues are manipulated during the process of developing the treatment. The rule defines homologous use as the "replacement, or supplementation of a recipient's cells or tissues with an HCT/P that performs the same basic function or functions in the recipient as in the donor"[10] and provides two definitions of minimal manipulation, one for structural tissue and the other for cells or nonstructural tissues. For structural tissue, minimal manipulation is defined as "processing that does not alter the original relevant characteristics of the tissue relating to the tissue's utility for reconstruction, repair, or replacement."[11]

For cells or nonstructural tissues, the 2001 regulation defines minimal manipulation as "processing that does not alter the relevant biological characteristics of cells or tissues."[12] In announcing the new rule, the FDA specifically noted that it did "not agree that the expansion of mesenchymal cells in culture or the use of growth factors to expand umbilical cord blood stem cells are minimal manipulation."[13] Thus, HCT/Ps that are more than minimally manipulated and used to perform other than their normal functions have to be tested in human clinical trials to determine their safety and effectiveness and be approved by the FDA prior to marketing them for clinical use.

FDA's Initial Enforcement Actions

In 2008, the FDA took action to enforce the 2001 regulation when it notified the Colorado company Regenerative Sciences that its autologous cultured cell product was subject to FDA approval as a drug under the FDCA and a biological product under the PHS Act. Regenerative Sciences was providing its product, the Regenexx Procedure, through an exclusive licensing agreement to an orthopedic clinic owned by Christopher Centeno and John Schultz. Centeno and Schultz were the majority shareholders of Regenerative Sciences, and Centeno was the medical director of the company. At the Centeno-Schultz Orthopedic Clinic, bone marrow was extracted from a patient's hip and a blood sample from the arm. These materials were sent to Regenerative Sciences's lab, where the patient's mesenchymal stem cells were isolated and cultured. The culturing process took one to two weeks, followed by quality assurance testing. When the processes were completed, patients returned to the orthopedic clinic to receive an infusion of the cultured mesenchymal stem cells at the injured area.[14]

The dispute between the FDA and Regenerative Sciences ended up in federal court, with Regenerative Sciences claiming that it was not manufacturing a drug or biological product under the FDCA or PHS Act and that Dr. Centeno was engaging in the practice of medicine, over which the FDA had no regulatory authority. Regenerative Sciences also claimed that its stem cell intervention was minimally manipulated and thus not subject to the FDA's 2001 regulation governing HCT/Ps. Centeno and others argued that the FDA should not require evidence of safety and effectiveness of autologous stem cell interventions from RCTs and that patients should be able to use their own cells without interference from the government. They also pointed out that patients would have to travel to other countries to get stem cell interventions if the FDA required these interventions to go through its lengthy drug development and approval process. Some patients and physicians also claimed that patients' testimonial reports and physicians' own experience treating patients should be an adequate base of evidence upon which to make decisions about the safety and effectiveness of stem cell interventions, even in the absence of reports in the medical literature of safety and effectiveness data derived from clinical trials.[15]

One patient who received a stem cell intervention as a so-called stem cell tourist was Dr. Stanley Jones, an orthopedic surgeon in Houston, Texas. In May 2010, Jones traveled to Japan to receive a stem cell intervention for his painful arthritis.[16] Convinced by his own experience that the intervention was therapeutically beneficial, Jones and a prominent Houston businessman formed the company Celltex Therapeutics to develop stem cell interventions for patients in the United States. The company obtained an exclusive license from the Korean company RNL-Bio to develop the interventions using RNL-Bio's proprietary stem cell culturing process. Over a three-week period, Celltex processed, cultured, and expanded patients' cells, which were then reinfused into patients as an autologous treatment.[17] The injections cost $20,000 to $30,000 and coordinating physicians reportedly received five hundred dollars from Celltex for each injection they administered.[18]

Texas governor Rick Perry, who became secretary of the U.S. Department of Energy in March 2017, was reported to be the first patient to receive a stem cell product from Celltex. A few weeks before announcing in the summer of 2011 that he was running for the U.S. presidency, Perry had back surgery that included injections of his cultured adult stem cells. In a presurgical procedure, Dr. Jones—who was also a friend of the governor—used liposuction to obtain fat cells from Perry's hip and sent the cells to Celltex's lab, where they were processed using RNL's culturing methods. Jones injected the processed cells into the governor's spine and bloodstream during the back surgery.[19]

Three weeks after receiving the stem cell intervention, Governor Perry—reportedly at the behest of Dr. Jones—asked the Texas Medical Board to adopt a new rule permitting physicians in Texas to offer patients stem cell interventions that were not approved by the FDA. Perry called on the Medical Board—whose members are gubernatorial appointees—to "recognize the revolutionary potential that adult stem cell research and therapies have on our nation's health, quality of life, and economy."[20] In April 2012, the Medical Board issued a rule that would permit only physicians to perform the procedure, require physicians to obtain prior approval by a review panel before offering patients a stem cell intervention, and require patients to give consent to receive the intervention.[21]

In November 2012, the FDA released a 483-page report of its on-site facility inspection of the Celltex lab, in which it listed 79 violations of processing and manufacturing requirements for HCT/Ps. Moreover, some patients claimed they were harmed by the company's stem cell intervention, and one media story reported that a patient had died after receiving the Celltex product.[22] The company was also mired in a legal dispute with RNL Bio involving financial issues, and by early 2013, Celltex announced that patients would only be able to receive the company's stem cell interventions from physicians in Mexico.[23] As of late 2017, Celltex advertised itself as a leading adult "stem cell bank" and was helping patients make arrangements to travel to Cancun, Mexico, to receive infusions or injections of their processed stem cells for regenerative therapy purposes.[24]

FDA Clarifies the Regulatory Approach

While the FDA was investigating Celltex, the litigation with Regenerative Sciences was winding its way through the federal courts. In February 2014, the U.S. Court of Appeals for the District of Columbia ruled that the FDA has the authority to regulate stem cell interventions and that doing so does not infringe on the right of the states to regulate within their jurisdiction the practice of medicine.[25] Later that year the agency issued three draft guidance documents regarding HCT/Ps: "Same Surgical Procedure Draft Guidance," "Minimal Manipulation Draft Guidance," and "Adipose Tissue Draft Guidance." In 2015 the agency issued the "Homologous Use Draft Guidance" along with an announcement that it would hold a one-day public hearing in April 2016 to discuss all four of the draft guidances. The FDA later said it was cancelling the April hearing in order hold a two-day hearing in September 2016, that it was opening a public comment period to obtain feedback about the draft guidances, and that it would hold a separate one-day meeting to focus on the science in developing HCT/Ps subject to the agency's regulatory requirements for premarket approval.[26] Unlike regulations, FDA guidance documents are nonbinding. Nonetheless, they give insight to the companies developing FDA-regulated products—and to the physicians who prescribe them and the patients who use them—what the agency's current thinking is about how it will interpret and enforce relevant regulations.

Overall, the draft guidances did not bring good news to product developers, physicians, and patients who wanted the FDA to relax its regulatory requirements for stem cell and other regenerative medicine interventions or to exempt some interventions from those requirements. Some physicians and patients contended that autologous stem cell interventions did not involve more than minimal manipulation of patients' cells. They also claimed that when patients received an infusion of their processed cells, it was part of the same surgical procedure to obtain the cells, even though the infusion might be administered days or weeks after their cells were harvested and sent to a processing site. In the "Same Surgical Procedure Draft Guidance," the FDA described a narrow set of circumstances under which establishments that manufacture human cellular or tissue-based products that meet certain criteria would be exempt from registering and listing with the agency.[27]

In the guidances on adipose tissue and minimal manipulation, the FDA also indicated its intent to use a narrow definition of minimal manipulation, which meant that many of the stem cell interventions that clinics in the United States were offering to patients would not be exempt from the agency's 2001 regulation for HCT/Ps. The agency said it considered "adipose tissue to be a structural tissue, with characteristics for reconstruction, repair, or replacement that relate to its utility to cushion and support the other tissues in the subcutaneous layer (subcutaneum) and skin."[28] and provided an example of a stem cell intervention involving the isolation of cells from structural tissue that would need premarket approval.

> A manufacturer recovers adipose tissue by tumescent liposuction and processes the adipose tissue to isolate cellular components, commonly referred to as stromal vascular fraction, which is considered a potential source of adipose-derived stromal/stem cells. The HCT/P generally is considered more than minimally manipulated because the processing breaks down and eliminates the structural components that provide cushioning and support, thereby altering the original relevant characteristics of the HCT/P relating to its utility for reconstruction, repair, or replacement.[29]

At the two-day public hearing to discuss the draft guidances, 93 speakers gave five-minute presentations. Fifty-four speakers were from for-profit and nonprofit entities—including companies developing and/or offering various types of HCT/Ps to patients—academic medical centers, tissue banks and organ transplant organizations, professional scientific/medical organizations, and patient advocacy groups. There also was a speaker from a law firm, a consulting firm, a think tank, and the California Institute for Regenerative Medicine, a state-funded institute that provides funding to organizations in the state conducting stem cell research. Thirty-nine speakers gave testimony in their capacity as individuals. Nearly all of these individuals—many of whom were patients and physicians—objected to the FDA regulating autologous stem cell interventions.[30]

There were however, researchers and health care providers at the public hearing who expressed support for the FDA's draft guidances and who raised concerns about lowering evidentiary standards for market entry of stem cell and other regenerative medicine interventions. Leigh Turner, a bioethics professor at the University Minnesota who supported the draft guidances, also criticized the FDA for not taking enforcement action against clinics offering patients unapproved stem cell interventions. In addition to publishing articles about unapproved stem cell clinics and the issue of stem cell tourism, Turner had been pressuring the FDA to investigate clinics in the United States that were marketing unapproved stem cell interventions. Three months before the public hearing, Turner published an article in which he and stem cell researcher Paul Knoepfler identified over 300 companies in the United States engaged in direct-to-consumer marketing of unapproved interventions promoted as treatments for a range of conditions, including orthopedic injuries, neurological disorders, cardiac disease, immunological and pulmonary disorders, spinal cord injuries, and cosmetic problems.[31]

Five days before the two-day public hearing, the FDA held a public workshop to discuss the scientific evidence for developing HCT/Ps subject to pre-market approval. Importantly, at that workshop, some scientists and others raised concerns about whether the stem cell treatments clinics and physicians were offering patients actually contained true stem cells rather than other types of human cells.[32] Since few of the interventions had been tested in clinical trials with the results published in relevant scientific and medical journals, it was difficult to know what kind of cells were used and to assess testimonial claims from physicians and patients of their safety and effectiveness.[33]

Stem Cells and Right-to-Try Laws

While the FDA was taking steps to develop a policy framework for regulating stem cell and other regenerative medicine interventions, policy initiatives to give patients access to unapproved medical interventions and to alter the evidentiary standards for claims of safety and effectiveness were being introduced in state legislatures and Congress. One way for patients to get access to unapproved drugs is to enroll in an FDA-approved clinical trial. Yet several barriers to enrollment prevent many people from getting access to investigational drugs being tested in clinical trials. For example, if one of the risks of an investigational drug is excessive bleeding, patients taking an anticlotting drug would probably not be permitted to enroll in the study. Another barrier to enrollment is when the trial is testing an intervention for a specific disease but the patient has a different disease and wants access to the intervention because of emerging evidence that it might be therapeutically effective for other indications.

Since the late 1990s, the FDA has facilitated "off-trial" access to investigational drugs for some patients under its "compassionate use" program. This program allows patients with a serious or life-threatening condition to apply—through a process their physician initiates—to the FDA and to drug manufacturers for access to a drug being tested in a clinical trial. Since 2010, the FDA has approved nearly all of the compassionate use requests that patients submitted. FDA approval for off-trial access to an investigational intervention does not, however, guarantee that patients will get the intervention, because the agency cannot force the drug company sponsoring the clinical trial to provide off-trial access. For various reasons, including concerns that providing off-trial access to investigational drugs will hinder them from enrolling enough patients in the trial, many companies decline to do so.[34]

Despite the fact that drug companies conducting clinical trials are the gatekeepers to off-trial access of their investigational intervention, the FDA was the target for many patients, free-market advocates, and others who had long argued that the agency was interfering with patients' right to use medical interventions they and their physician decided were best for them. The Goldwater Institute, a libertarian research and advocacy organization, has led the nationwide effort for passage of state and federal laws designed to permit patients to bypass the FDA's requirements for off-trial access to investigational interventions. Proponents of these "right-to-try" laws claim that seriously ill patients have a right to investigational drugs for which there is limited evidence about their safety and effectiveness and that the government should not prohibit them from getting access to them.[35] When he introduced the Compassionate Freedom of Choice Act in 2014 in the U.S. House of Representatives, Rep. Morgan Griffith (R-VA) asked why the FDA should have to approve off-label access to an investigational intervention when a patient was aware of the intervention's potential risks, obtained approval from a physician, and was willing to pay out of pocket for the intervention. "The FDA," said Griffith, "was created to protect us from harmful drugs. If I'm dying anyway, shouldn't I have the freedom to decide if the risk is worth it?"[36]

Right-to-Try in the States

In 2014, Colorado became the first state to pass a right-to-try law, and by December 2017, 37 states had enacted similar laws. The laws differ in their details, but they typically permit patients to bypass the FDA's requirement that (1) an institutional review board (IRB) with jurisdiction over research with human subjects must approve the request for access to the intervention being tested in a trial at that institution, and (2) the patient's physician must submit data to the agency about the outcome of the patient's use of the intervention.[37] Soon after the Colorado legislature passed its right-to-try law, the stem cell company Neuralstem said it was hoping to use the new law to give patients with amyotrophic lateral sclerosis (ALS) access to the stem cell interventions it was testing in phase II clinical trials. At that time, Neuralstem's chief executive, I. Richard Garr, was the chair of the Goldwater Institute's Right to Try National Advisory Council.[38]

Although Texas already had a right-to-try law, in 2017 Governor Greg Abbott signed a law that specifically gives patients off-trial access to an investigational stem cell treatment, defined as "an adult stem cell treatment that is under investigation in a clinical trial and being administered to human participants in that trial and has not yet been approved for general use" by the FDA.[39] Patients with certain severe chronic diseases or terminal illnesses are eligible for access to an investigational stem cell treatment when certain conditions are met: the patient's physician (1) attests that the patient has a severe chronic disease or terminal illness as defined in the statute; (2) consults with the patient in determining that all FDA-approved treatment options "are unavailable or unlikely to alleviate the significant impairment or severe pain associated with the severe chronic disease or terminal illness; and (3) recommends or prescribes in writing "that the patient use a specific class of investigational stem cell treatment." The law prohibits the Texas Medical Board from revoking, failing to renew, suspending, or taking any actions against a physician's license solely because the physician recommended that an eligible patient have access to the investigational stem cell treatment, on condition that the physician's recommendations or medical care reflect the standard of care and comply with the provisions of the right-to-try law. Moreover, the law prohibits patients who believe they were harmed by an investigational stem cell intervention they received pursuant to the law to sue the developer of the intervention or any other person or entity involved in their care.

As with the more general right-to-try laws, the Texas stem cell treatment right-to-try law does not require a drug company to provide patients with off-trial access to the investigational intervention. Moreover, the bill does not say whether the clinical trial assessing an investigational intervention has to be an FDA-approved trial or if physicians can call their office-based study in which they collect outcomes data from patients a clinical trial. And the legislature left it to the commissioner of the state's Health and Human Services Commission to determine what medical conditions meet the definition of a chronic disease or terminal condition.

The Texas stem cell treatment right-to-try law went into effect September 1, 2017, with the stipulation that as soon as practicable after its effective date, the executive commissioner of the state's Health and Human Services Commission will adopt rules necessary for its implementation. According to news reports, the commission is expected to work with the state medical board to develop rules mandating that physicians provide a stem cell intervention in an ambulatory center, a hospital, or a medical school[40] and that oversight by IRB will be required.[41]

Right-to-Try in Congress

Several right-to-try bills have also been introduced in Congress. In August 2017, the Senate approved by unanimous consent S. 204, which was sponsored by Sen. Ron Johnson (R-WI). The proposed "Trickett Wendler, Frank Mongiello, Jordan McLinn, and Matthew Bellina Right to Try Act of 2017"[42] would amend the FDCA to give patients with a life-threatening disease or condition off-trial access to certain investigational drugs: those for which a phase I safety trial has been completed and have moved into a later-stage

FDA-approved trial to establish their effectiveness. Eligible patients would be permitted to bypass the FDA's compassionate use program by letting them go directly to the drug company testing the investigational drug after their physician certifies they have exhausted all other treatment options. Although some public health advocates, representatives of the drug industry, and officials at the FDA raised concerns about the initial version that permitted patients to bypass getting approval from their physician and the FDA, Senator Johnson threatened to hold up a five-year reauthorization of the FDA's user fee programs if the Senate refused to pass the bill. The revisions that led to its passage in the Senate included requiring that drug companies provide the FDA with reports of safety events from off-trial access and forbidding them from charging patients for more than the cost of production for the investigational drug.[43]

At a hearing on the bill that the House Subcommittee on Energy and Commerce held on October 3, 2017, FDA commissioner Scott Gottlieb described the agency's program for patient access to investigational interventions. With regard to the proposed right-to-try bill, Gottlieb recommended that Congress narrow the eligibility from patients facing a "life-threatening disease or condition" to "terminal illness." He suggested this change would be consistent with the intent of most proponents of right-to-try initiatives. Gottlieb also pointed out the need for a clear definition of "terminal illness" and said the FDA recommended defining the term as "a stage of disease in which there is a reasonable likelihood that death will occur within a matter of months."[44] In addition to taking the position that "terminal illness" be narrowly defined, Gottlieb also took the opportunity to remind committee members of the importance of the clinical trials process for obtaining evidence about whether medical technologies are safe and if they work. Said Gottlieb,

> The clinical trials process is crucial to the development of innovative new medical products that can improve or save patients' lives. Adequate policies and processes must be in place to appropriately balance individual patients' needs for access to investigational therapies while recognizing the importance of maintaining a rigorous clinical trial paradigm for testing investigational products to demonstrate safety and efficacy.[45]

According to one news report, the bill was stalled in the House partly in response to concerns Gottlieb raised at the hearing and because pharmaceutical companies were worried their drug approval applications to the FDA could be jeopardized if they provided their investigational drugs to patients off trial.[46] The political heat to pass the bill became more intense after Vice President Pence and President Trump joined the chorus of supporters. Pence tweeted on January 18, 2018, "Let's get this DONE," and mentioned a meeting he had that week with Gottlieb to find a way to move the bill forward.[47]

And in his first State of the Union address on January 30, President Trump said, "It is time for the Congress to give [people who are terminally ill] the right to try."[48] On May 30, 2018, President Trump signed a right-to-try law that had been adopted by Congress on May 22nd.

Regenerative Medicine and the 21st Century Cures Act

Congress took specific aim at the FDA's regulation of stem cell and other regenerative medicine interventions when it passed the 21st Century Cures Act in late 2016. First introduced in the House in May 2015 by Representatives Fred Upton (R-MI) and Diana DeGette (D-CO), the Cures Act was promoted as a bipartisan effort to accelerate the pace at which medical treatments and cures would reach patients and "to ensure we are taking full advantage of the advances this country has made in science and technology and use these resources to keep America as the innovation capital of the world."[49] The initiative was the brainchild of Upton, who said he was compelled to act after meeting children with rare diseases who had few therapeutic options.[50]

Significantly, the final version of the bill President Obama signed contained provisions in section 3033, "Accelerated Approval for Regenerative Advanced Therapies," that were not in the initial version Upton and DeGette introduced in 2015. Some of the new provisions were revised provisions of the proposed "Reliable and Effective Growth for Regenerative Health Options that Improve Wellness (REGROW) Act" that Senator Kirk (R-IL) introduced in the Senate (S. 2689) on March 16, 2016 and Representative Mike Coffman (R-CO) introduced the same day in the House (H.R. 4762). As a former stroke patient, Kirk said he introduced the REGROW Act so that other stroke patients and patients with Alzheimer's, Parkinson's, and diabetes could get faster access to promising stem cell interventions.[51]

The proposed REGROW Act would have permitted the FDA to grant conditional approval to a cellular therapeutic product without data from phase II or phase III trials if the product developer provided preliminary clinical evidence showing safety and a reasonable expectation of effectiveness. To be eligible for conditional approval, a cell or tissue product had to comprise adult cells or tissues that were minimally manipulated for a nonhomologous use, or more than minimally manipulated for a homologous or nonhomologous use—but not genetically modified. The product also had to be "produced exclusively for a use that performs, or helps achieve or restore, the same, or similar, function in the recipient as in the donor."[52] To obtain FDA approval for continued use of the product after a five-year conditional approval period, the manufacturer would have to submit to the agency annual reports that include adverse events data and other information typically required for FDA-approved biological products.

Conflicting Interest Group Positions

Many patient advocacy organizations and stem cell companies supported the REGROW Act, including a wealthy Texas entrepreneur who owned at least one regenerative medicine company and contributed millions of dollars to Republican super PACs—political action committees that are legally permitted to raise unlimited amounts of money from corporations, unions, and individuals to spend on state and federal elections.[53] The bill also garnered strong support from the Bipartisan Policy Center—a Washington, DC think tank formed in 2007 by four former U.S. Senate majority leaders (two Republicans and two Democrats). The Center released a policy paper in December 2015, in which it contended that cell products should be subject to different FDA review and approval standards than pharmaceutical drugs, that current regulatory standards posed a barrier to patients using their own cells, and that once cell therapies are shown to be safe, the FDA should accelerate their market entry, even if they were still being assessed for effectiveness in early-phase clinical trials.[54]

Yet there were dissenting voices in the patient advocacy and product development communities regarding the proposed bill. A coalition of ten patient advocacy groups sent a letter to Senator Kirk expressing concerns that the REGROW Act would lower the FDA's evidentiary standards for market approval of regenerative medicine interventions and that once the FDA granted conditional approval, it would be difficult for the agency to withdraw the interventions from the market if postmarketing data revealed they were unsafe or ineffective. The groups also noted that the FDA already had several pathways for accelerating the drug development and approval process. The organizations that signed the letter included the Cystic Fibrosis Foundation, Friedreich's Ataxia Research Alliance, Friends of Cancer Research, Global Genes, Michael J. Fox Foundation for Parkinson's Research, Myotonic Dystrophy Foundation, National MS Society, National Organization for Rare Disorders, National Patient Advocate Foundation, and the Prevent Cancer Foundation.[55]

Opposition to the REGROW Act also came from two major advocacy organizations for regenerative medicine and stem cell research: the Alliance for Regenerative Medicine and the International Society for Stem Cell Research. Members of both of the organizations included scientists and representatives from pharmaceutical and biotech companies. In a letter to Senator Kirk, the Alliance for Regenerative Medicine said that "by calling into question whether Phase III trials should ever be required to receive this new type of 'conditional approval' status," the REGROW Act "potentially allows products on the market without necessary testing we believe to be required for complex products such as autologous cell therapies."[56] And the International Society for Stem Cell Research pointed out that "If new medical products can be sold to patients before their effectiveness is rigorously demonstrated, the government, private healthcare systems, and insurers may be compelled to reimburse the costs of new treatments without knowing whether they work."[57]

From REGROW to the Cures Act

The REGROW Act never reached a committee vote in the House or the Senate. Even so, a revised version of several provisions found their way into the Cures Act. Significantly, Section 3033 created a designation the FDA can give certain stem cell and regenerative medicine interventions to qualify for the agency's existing expedited approval programs. To qualify for a "regenerative medicine advanced therapy" (RMAT) designation, a drug must be (1) a cell therapy, therapeutic tissue engineering product, human cell and tissue product, or combination product using any such therapies or products (unless solely under provisions of the PHS); (2) "intended to treat, modify, reverse, or cure a serious or life-threatening disease or condition; and 3) have the potential "to address unmet medical needs for such disease or condition" based on preliminary clinical evidence.[58]

The RMAT designation does not guarantee the FDA will grant market approval for the product. However, unlike drugs without the RMAT designation that qualify for the agency's expedited approval pathways, RMAT products approved through those pathways can meet postapproval requirements with data derived from sources other than standard RCTs. To fulfill postapproval requirements, the product developer is required to provide the FDA with data about safety and effectiveness from various sources of "real world evidence," including patient registries, electronic medical records, larger confirmatory data sets, or postapproval monitoring of patients who were treated with the intervention before the FDA approved it for market entry.

The New Political and Regulatory Landscape

Scientists conducting studies using human cells and tissues and companies in the regenerative medicine product sector are eager to get their products to patients as fast as possible. Yet some of these stakeholders raised concerns that policy initiatives like the proposed REGROW Act went too far in changing the FDA's regulatory authority over regenerative medicine interventions and in altering the evidentiary standards of safety and effectiveness. It was not lost on many of these stakeholders that policy initiatives to accelerate access to untested and unapproved stem cell and other regenerative medicine interventions or to relax evidentiary standards of safety and effectiveness are in tension with the goal of achieving commercial success for their products. As the chair of the Alliance for Regenerative Medicine pointed out when the REGROW Act was proposed, "What we don't need at this point are products that go onto the market under some conditional approval process that aren't rigorously tested and could truly compromise the whole industry."[59]

Thus, some medical experts and leaders from the pharmaceutical industry were alarmed when President Trump announced soon after he assumed the presidency that he would deregulate the FDA by eliminating between 75 and 80 percent of the agency's regulations and streamlining the drug approval process.[60] Industry executives and others also raised concerns about potential candidates he was considering to be commissioner of the FDA, particularly Jim O'Neill, who believes that once phase I trials indicate that drugs are safe, drug companies should not have to test for effectiveness in additional clinical trials as a condition of obtaining premarket approval. O'Neill, a libertarian who was a former official at HHS, said that people should be able to start using drugs shown to be safe "at their own risk," with effectiveness evidence to come after market approval.[61]

The president eventually nominated Scott Gottlieb, MD, a former FDA deputy commissioner with strong ties to industry resulting from his consultant work with many pharmaceutical companies. Gottlieb had previously worked at the agency as deputy commissioner for medical and scientific affairs. According to one media report, Gottlieb was viewed as someone who would preserve the FDA's basic role of ensuring that drugs gaining market entry are safe and effective, not as someone who wanted to dismantle the FDA. Nonetheless, he was also described as someone who likely would "try shaking it up in significant ways."[62] Moreover, Gottlieb had been critical of the FDA's approach to regulating stem cell interventions and questioned whether safety and effectiveness data had to come from RCTs. In a policy paper he coauthored while a fellow at the American Enterprise Institute, Gottlieb asked how a large-scale RCT could be conducted and "ensure consistency from one use of a drug to another, where the 'drug' is really a medical procedure that must vary from one patient to the next because it involves their own unique cells?" And echoing the claims of others who objected to the FDA's regulatory stance over stem cell interventions, he said the agency's approach "can't be readily satisfied when it comes to treatments that are personalized to individual patients."[63]

Yet, in August 2017—three months after he was sworn in as the FDA's 23rd commissioner—Gottlieb issued a statement suggesting that under his helm, the agency would continue to require FDA premarket approval for some stem cell interventions.

Gottlieb's First Steps

Commissioner Gottlieb announced in August 2017 that the FDA was developing "new policy and enforcement efforts to ensure proper oversight of stem cell therapies and regenerative medicine."[64] Gottlieb noted that stem cell therapies "hold significant promise for transformative and potentially curative treatments for some of humanity's most troubling and intractable maladies." But the entire field of regenerative medicine was at risk, he said, if

> bad actors are able to make hollow claims and market unsafe science. In such an environment a select few, often motivated by greed without regard to responsible patient care, are able to promote unproven, clearly illegal, and often expensive treatments that offer little hope, and, even worse, may pose significant risks to the health and safety of vulnerable patients. These so-called treatments run afoul of the FDA's legal and regulatory framework governing this new field.[65]

Gottlieb also announced that in the fall of 2017, the FDA would roll out a "comprehensive policy framework that will more clearly describe the rules of the road for this new field" and that the agency had begun to step up its enforcement activities to prevent the manufacturing and use of stem cell interventions for which the FDA had not granted premarket approval.[66] In a warning letter dated August 24, 2017, the agency informed a Florida clinic, U.S. Stem Cell Clinic, that the stem cell intervention it was providing as a treatment for various diseases, including Parkinson's disease, ALS, rheumatoid arthritis, and chronic obstructive pulmonary disease did not meet the agency's regulatory requirements as a drug pursuant to the FDCA, as a biological product pursuant to the PHS, or as HCT/Ps pursuant to the agency's regulations issued in 2001 governing these products.[67]

The agency also announced that it had enlisted help from the U.S. Marshal service to seize samples of the smallpox vaccine from a company in California that was using the vaccine to develop an autologous stem cell intervention. The company, StemImmune, processed stem cells derived from patients' body fat (stromal vascular fraction) with a small amount of the vaccine, then sent the processed cells to a clinic where each patient's processed cells were injected into their cancerous tumors. According to the FDA, the treatment posed potentially dangerous harms, "including myocarditis and pericarditis (inflammation and swelling of the heart and surrounding tissues)" to cancer patients who may have compromised immune systems.[68]

FDA's New Policy Framework

As promised, the FDA announced its new comprehensive regenerative medicine policy framework in November 2017. The agency issued two draft guidance documents and two final guidance documents describing plans to implement various provisions of the Cures Act, including the RMAT designation. Commissioner Gottlieb said the goal of the new policy framework was to "advance a modern, efficient and least burdensome framework that recognizes the breakneck speed of advancement in the products we're being asked to evaluate, while ensuring patient safety." Embedded in the framework, he said, are proposed novel and modern approaches to regulation—including innovative clinical trial designs—that would help the FDA adapt its "regulatory model to meet the revolutionary nature of the products we're being asked to evaluate."[69]

The final guidance documents on HCT/Ps the FDA issued in November 2017 indicate that the agency has not drastically altered the position it laid out in the draft guidances issued in 2014 and 2015. The agency noted that it had received many inquiries from manufacturers about whether their HCT/Ps meet the criteria for minimal manipulation and/or homologous use, and provided a flowchart in one of the final guidance documents for how to apply the criteria.[70] It explained that when applying the minimal manipulation criterion, the first step is to determine whether the HCT/P is structural or cellular/nonstructural. And the agency did not alter its position that adipose tissue is a structural tissue for the purpose of applying the HCT/P regulatory framework. This means that many of the unapproved types of stem cell interventions that clinics and physicians in the United States are offering patients are likely subject to FDA's premarket approval requirements. In the final guidance on minimal manipulation and homologous use, the FDA provided such an example:

> Example 11-1: Original relevant characteristics of adipose tissue relating to its utility to provide cushioning and support generally include its bulk and lipid storage capacity. A manufacturer processes adipose tissue by removing the cells, which leaves the decellularized extracellular matrix portion of the HCT/P. The HCT/P generally is considered more than minimally manipulated because the processing alters the original relevant characteristics of the HCT/P relating to its utility to provide cushioning and support.[71]

Later in the final guidance, the agency explained that by isolating cells from structural tissue, "the definition of minimal manipulation for structural tissue applies, regardless of the method used to isolate the cells. This is because the assessment of whether the HCT/P is a structural tissue or cellular/nonstructural tissue is based on the characteristics of the HCT/P as it exists in the donor, prior to recovery and any processing that takes place." The example provided further clarified this position:

> Example 14-1: Original relevant characteristics of adipose tissue relating to its utility to provide cushioning and support generally include its bulk and lipid storage capacity. A manufacturer recovers adipose tissue by tumescent liposuction and processes (e.g., enzymatically digests, mechanically

disrupts, etc.) the adipose tissue to isolate cellular components (with or without subsequent cell culture or expansion), commonly referred to as stromal vascular fraction, which is considered a potential source of adipose-derived stromal/stem cells. The definition of minimal manipulation for structural tissue applies.[72]

The FDA explained that it generally considered the HCT/P in this example to be "more than minimally manipulated because the processing breaks down and eliminates the adipocytes and the surrounding structural components that provide cushioning and support, thereby altering the original relevant characteristics of the HCT/P relating to its utility for reconstruction, repair, or replacement."[73]

Conclusion

The FDA announced its new regulatory framework governing stem cell and other regenerative medicine interventions after a decade-long dispute about the "path to the clinic" for these types of interventions. Demands for patients' access to unapproved stem cell interventions could be heard in the debate over so-called right-to-try laws that have been introduced in Congress and that, as of April 2018, 40 states have enacted. And accelerating patient access to stem cell and other regenerative medicine interventions was the motivation for Section 3033 of the Cures Act that created the RMAT designation.

In his statement announcing the agency's new policy for regenerative medicine products, Commissioner Gottlieb acknowledged that product developers will need time to determine whether their stem cell and other regenerative medicine interventions require FDA approval, and if they do, to consult with the FDA about submitting an application for marketing authorization.[74] The final guidance on minimal manipulation and homologous use specifies that for the first 36 months following issuance of the guidance, the FDA will exercise enforcement discretion over FDA-regulated HCT/Ps intended for autologous use that physicians provide to their patients, as long as no safety concerns from clinical use are reported or no potential safety concerns are identified.

Since Turner and Knoepfler had reported a year earlier that at least 570 clinics throughout the country were offering stem cell interventions,[75] some commentators wondered if the FDA's enforcement discretion approach was a signal to those clinics that the agency would not be aggressively investigating whether the interventions required premarket approval. Some also suggested that the agency lacked the resources to investigate so many clinics, and that the three-year discretionary enforcement period was a way to give product developers a chance to apply for premarket approval if their products they were already marketing to physicians and patients needed such approval under the new regulatory framework. In response to concerns that the FDA was backing off from undertaking investigations and enforcement actions, an FDA spokesperson said the agency would not exercise enforcement discretion when HCT/Ps pose a significant safety concern.[76] It remains to be seen whether the FDA has the resources—and the political will—to follow through with its risk-based approach to enforce its regulatory framework governing market entry of stem cell and regenerative medicine interventions.

Importantly, some stem cell and other regenerative medicine interventions that meet the criteria in the Cures Act for the RMAT designation could eventually be approved by the FDA through an accelerated approval pathway. This means that, as is the case for some traditional pharmaceutical drugs, HCT/Ps given the RMAT designation might obtain market approval on the basis of safety and effectiveness evidence from a small number of clinical trials with few patient-participants, and from surrogate or intermediate end points. What is unknown at this time is whether the FDA will grant market approval to these products with data obtained from sources other than RCTs, and whether the agency will—as it did with Avastin—closely monitor the postmarketing use of RMAT-designated interventions and be willing to withdraw marketing approval if the products pose serious harm to patients. One thing is certain, however: the FDA's new policy framework governing stem cell and other regenerative medicine interventions has not resolved the debate over evidentiary standards of safety and effectiveness that should be met before patients have access to such interventions.

Conclusion: The 21st Century Cures Act and the Future of Health Technology Assessment

The regulatory system requiring FDA market approval for certain medical technologies was established in response to incidents of drugs that harmed and killed people, with the goal of protecting individual patients and the public from harmful and ineffective products. "Patient tragedy" and "public health protection" narratives were the central policy frames for the Pure Food and Drug Act of 1906; the Federal Food, Drug, and Cosmetic Act of 1938; and the 1962 Kefauver-Harris Drug Amendments to the FDCA, all of which promoted government regulation of the market entry of pharmaceutical drugs. By the 1980s, these narratives—which emerged in response to the "absence of a regulatory sentry" in the early 20th century to keep unsafe drugs away from patients[1]—lost their salience as the dominant policy frame for regulating market entry of new medical technologies. New patient tragedy narratives emerged that aligned with free market and neoliberal ideologies about the role of government in regulating new medical technologies: that patients are harmed by not getting access to medical technologies because the FDA's approval process takes too long and that the agency's evidentiary standards for safety and effectiveness are too high. Accompanying this new patient tragedy narrative was a different tragedy narrative: that the FDA's outdated and slow drug approval process and evidentiary standards were harming medical product innovation and the country's reputation as a global leader in the medical product sector.

Rather than deregulating the FDA in the way some free market advocates have envisioned—such as transferring the drug evaluation and approval process to the private sector[2]—in the post-thalidomide era, Congress recalibrated the regulatory approach by instructing the FDA to expedite the drug development and review process, and specifically with the 21st Century Cures Act, to develop programs to incorporate the use of evidence of safety and effectiveness from various sources of data. In addition to the provisions regarding the RMAT designation for certain HCT/Ps, the Cures Act includes provisions instructing the FDA to (1) issue guidance addressing the use of complex adaptive and other novel trial designs and how trials with such designs will satisfy the substantial evidence standard for premarket approval and (2) establish a program to evaluate the potential use of real-world evidence (RWE), defined as "data regarding the usage, or the potential benefits or risks, of a drug derived from sources other than randomized clinical trials."[3]

This push for loosening evidentiary standards and speeding the time it takes to bring some new technologies to the market, however, is not the only narrative competing in the policy arena. Another narrative emphasizes the need for better, more consistent evidence about the use of medical technologies and the practice of medicine. Since the late 1970s, when John Wennberg, Robert Brook, and other pioneers in health-services research started documenting unexplained variations in the use of health care services, there has been a desire to develop a stronger evidence base for health care decision making and to encourage the more appropriate use of technology. While some of the individuals and groups pushing for the deregulation of medical technology reject the science on which our longstanding regulatory regimens are based, it would be inaccurate and unfair to suggest everyone pushing for faster access to cures is opposed to the use of evidence. But there is no question that there are important disagreements about what counts as evidence, what thresholds of evidence are appropriate for allowing drugs and devices on the market, and what criteria payers should use when deciding whether to cover medical technologies. These tensions are illustrated well by the cases in this book. Equally important, disagreements about these ideas are often linked closely with economic and organizational interests, party affiliations, and ideological perspectives on the appropriate role of government. Epistemological disagreements matter, but they cannot be separated neatly from factors that are often labeled, pejoratively, as "politics." Our goal is not to identify the independent contributions of interest group struggles, partisan fights about the size of government, or disagreements about the validity of surrogate end points (or other sources of scientific disagreement) but to illustrate how these factors combine to shape the public debates about the value of medical technology.

What "counts" as evidence in evaluating the risks and benefits of new medical technologies? How much evidence, and from what "evidence sources," about a technology's risks and benefits is needed before patients can get access to that technology at the point of care and before public and private insurers should pay for it? Scholars of science and technology studies have shown that epistemological questions are not free of values and interests of the actors involved in scientific inquiry and evaluation of evidence.[4] These and other scholars have drawn attention to how scientific questions are constructed, by whom, and for what purposes; how boundaries are constructed to legitimate some forms of inquiry and data as "scientific," and others as "nonscience" or "pseudoscience";[5] how methods for gathering information affect what type and amount of information is captured; and how methods for analyzing the information collected influence knowledge claims about the focus of the inquiry.[6]

Studies of disputes about health technology assessment in regulatory, payer, and clinical settings also show that competing stakeholders bring to those disputes different values and interests about patient choice, physician autonomy, risk assessment, and government intervention in medicine and technology assessment.[7] A central theme in many evidence disputes is the "risk versus risk dilemma"—the risk of approving a drug or device that has serious side effects versus the risk of not approving it and some patients not getting a technology that might have therapeutic benefit for them. Patients and patient advocacy organizations that value accelerated access may consider risks of harm from a technology as a risk worth taking, often putting them at odds with regulators who make decisions about patient access through the lens of population-based risk-benefit considerations.[8]

Disputes about evidentiary standards for new biomedical technologies are also framed by the broader political economy in which technologies are evaluated. The translation and commercialization of new technologies have significant implications for generating the "appetite for innovation" needed to create new technologies that address patients' prevention, diagnostic, and treatment needs.[9] Echoing the idea behind Charles Lindblom's "privileged position of business" argument,[10] policy decisions from the perspective of economization are justified in terms of their effects on the economy.[11] Calls for lowering evidentiary standards when allowing new health technologies on the market or when using public dollars to purchase these technologies may have greater resonance when proponents emphasize the contributions of technology innovation to economic growth—or when they suggest that strict regulatory standards may lead to a loss of jobs to countries with lower standards. Echoes of these arguments are found in all of the cases in this book that involve some effort to restrict medical technologies.

On another level, debates "made epistemological"[12] often mask underlying political disputes.[13] As our cases illustrate, science and health policy disputes in the United States are frequently caught up in ideological divides about science and evidence[14] and in the maelstrom of partisan electoral politics, where short-term responses to complex problems have become the norm.[15] Recent studies suggest that the "core beliefs about science and society shape public opinion" about particular scientific disputes.[16] Other studies emphasize the extent to which debates about science are influenced by the degree to which they are viewed through a partisan or ideological lens.[17] For example, one study found that conservatives are more likely than liberals to trust scientists who develop new technologies but less likely than liberals to trust scientists who focus on the "environmental and public health impacts of economic production."[18] Commenting on the recent FDA decision to withdraw Avastin's authorization for advanced breast cancer, Carpenter argues that "the scientific debate over Avastin has been imbued with the ideological overtones of a debate over rationing and the role of regulation in American society."[19] Ideological overtones have also been present in debates about whether CMS will pay for Medicare patients to get access to medical technologies. As Gillick notes, "CMS is under pressure from Congress to make innovations available to the public as quickly as possible. The notion of imposing limits is seen as rationing, which is widely held to be anathema on the Hill."[20]

The Importance of Framing in Scientific Disputes

As many scholars in science and technology studies and political science have pointed out, values about science, risks and benefits of medical technologies—and the role of the state in regulating market entry of those technologies—influences what information "counts" for making claims about safety and effectiveness.[21] The values that people hold influence how they frame choices about competing policy approaches to medical technology. Scholars have also shown that politics is a "battle over ideas, and the ability to successfully control the dominant metaphors, the boundaries of categories, and the meanings of abstract, contested concepts, in order to persuade others."[22] In this book, we have examined the "policy frames" of key stakeholders involved in these evidence disputes. According to Schön and Rein, a policy frame is "a way of selecting, interpreting, and organizing information to construct a policy argument."[23] Identifying and understanding what value judgments stakeholders bring to their assessment of scientific facts helps us understand competing perspectives on how to regulate and whether to pay for medical technologies. Indeed, learning about the presumptive world of policymakers and other policy stakeholders is important for understanding what issues reach the policy agenda, how problems are defined, and how solutions are valued.

It is critical to understand different perspectives about the clinical utility of medical technologies. Debates about how to define clinical utility are central to disagreements about the evidentiary standards for patient access to new medical technologies. For example, CMS and many private payers do not cover the use of PET scans combined with radiopharmaceutical products (amyloid PET imaging) to identify amyloid plaque in patients with cognitive impairments being diagnosed for possible Alzheimer's disease. Payers question the clinical utility of the information obtained from amyloid PET imaging, claiming that insufficient evidence about the information leads to clinical management decisions that improve patient health outcomes. Yet many researchers, clinicians, representatives from industry, imaging associations, patients, and patient advocacy groups claim there is "value in knowing" that a patient has amyloid plaque in his or her brain, and thus the clinical utility of imaging information should be defined broadly.

The fight over mammography screening raised similar concerns. Are recommendations for limiting the use of mammography screening an effort to protect women from unnecessary suffering and avoid wasting limited resources, or is this an example of unwarranted rationing in which heartless bureaucrats value cost savings over the lives of women? There is obviously a factual dimension to this debate, but an appeal to facts alone cannot mediate the dispute. Even if we reach an agreement about the percentage of false positives associated with regular mammography screening among women age 40 to 49, this will not tell us what the policy or clinical response to such evidence ought to be. Better evidence about whether surrogate indicators, like progression-free survival, are related to overall survival or other measures designed to capture quality of life may help settle disputes about the use of drugs like Avastin, but there are still likely to be disagreements about the value placed on the surrogate end point itself.

Who Should Have the Power to Decide?

Some patients claim that their personal perception of therapeutic effectiveness—their "experiential evidence"—along with similar claims from other patients is valid and reliable evidence that justifies unfettered access to medical technologies that have not been evaluated in traditional clinical trials or for which there is incomplete trial data regarding safety and effectiveness.[24] For these patients, the answer to the "risk-versus-risk dilemma" is clear: getting access sooner rather than later to a medical technology that could help them but may have serious side effects is a risk worth taking, rather than the risk of missing an opportunity for potential therapeutic benefit by waiting for clinical trials data about safety and effectiveness.

For other proponents of unfettered patient access to medical technologies, the fundamental issue is about the role of the state in regulating market entry of medical technologies. Free-market advocates who want few regulatory controls over the market entry of medical technologies may agree with patients who say their experiential evidence is sufficient for access to medical technologies, but their push for relaxing or eliminating state regulations comes from an ideological stance that privileges freedom from state intervention above other justifications.

Several of the cases also revealed that some stakeholders—including product developers—favored altering the regulatory requirements for market entry of medical technologies but not eliminating all of those requirements. Indeed, regulations often provide advantages to industry that outweigh the disadvantages. Product developers will get their interventions to the market faster under the accelerated approval pathway for some drugs—and the new RMAT designation for HCT/Ps—but regulatory standards still govern how they must obtain valid and reliable safety and effectiveness data.

Complex Coalitions and Competition among Powerful Interest Groups

Patient advocacy groups often play an important role in debates about medical technology, but there often is no uniform advocacy position within and across all stakeholder groups, including within specific patient populations and across patient advocacy organizations. In media accounts of disputes about access to medical technologies—and at FDA public hearings—the dominant voices are often the "urgency narratives" of patients pushing for access or large advocacy organizations with corporate connections that have a stake in continuing to push a particular medical technology.[25] Yet as the Avastin and stem cell cases revealed, not all patients and advocacy organizations agree with those in favor of greater risk-taking when the evidence base regarding safety and effectiveness is incomplete or in dispute. And in the disputes about mammography screening, amyloid PET imaging, Avastin and stem cell therapies, there was disagreement among physicians, professional specialty groups, and organizations conducting technology assessments about the risks and benefits of these medical technologies and their value to the relevant patient populations. In the case of the new hepatitis C drugs, there is broad agreement among physicians and patient groups about the effectiveness of the drugs but conflicts with private and public payers over whether there is an obligation to pay for them, and conflicts between the pharmaceutical industry—and just about everyone else—over how much they are worth.

Paying for Technology and Disagreements about Public Priorities

The cases also reveal that FDA approval for market entry is no guarantee that public and private insurers will pay for the technology. Insurers may want to see different outcomes data than what the FDA reviewed for granting market approval, and their evidentiary bar for showing safety and effectiveness may be higher than that needed for FDA approval. For the amyloid PET imaging test, CMS argued that meeting the FDA's evidentiary standards—showing that when used with a PET scan, the radiopharmaceutical florbetapir identified amyloid plaque in a living brain—was not the same as showing that physicians' use of this information led to improved health outcomes for their relevant patients.

Although the cost issue was explicit only in the hepatitis C case, it was an undercurrent in all of the cases. For example, CMS is prohibited from taking cost into consideration when making coverage decisions, though some commentators contend that in several NCDs, the agency referred to and even used evidence about the cost-effectiveness of the technology under review.[26] Of note is that the 2008 Medicare Improvements for Patients and Providers Act contains language that could be interpreted as permitting CMS to explicitly consider cost-effectiveness information when it is making a decision about whether to cover a preventive service.[27] Yet when Congress passed the ACA, the bill included provisions prohibiting Medicare "from using a specific threshold for a cost per [quality-adjusted life year] in making reimbursement and coverage decisions" and limiting the way the program can use results from comparative-effectiveness research in making coverage decisions.[28]

Questions about the value of medical interventions in relation to their cost may take on greater significance in the 21st Cures era, as the FDA approves more drugs and biologics on the basis of evidence from early-phase RCTs with a few patients who received the investigational intervention, or from alternative sources of data that may have been collected with less precise rigor than would be the case with RCTs. Accelerated approval of Exondys 51 to treat Duchenne muscular dystrophy, a disease that causes muscles to deteriorate, is a recent example. FDA commissioner Robert Calif approved the drug through the accelerated-approval pathway, against the recommendation of agency experts who did not think the limited clinical trials data showed therapeutic effectiveness. The disease affects primarily young boys, most of whom die before they turn 30 years old. Parents of these patients have fought with several insurance companies that refuse to pay for the treatment, on the grounds that there is insufficient evidence from the accelerated-approval process that the drug helps protect muscle cells from deteriorating. The company that developed the drug says it will cost patients on average about $300,000 a year, though one news report says the cost could go as high as $1 million a year.[29] As *New York Times* reporter Katie Thomas points out, "The story of Exondys 51 raises complex and emotionally charged questions about what happens when the F.D.A. approves an expensive drug based on a lower bar of proof. In practice, health insurers have taken over as gatekeeper in determining who will get the drug."[30]

Another example that has implications for HCT/Ps the FDA will eventually approve under the RMAT designation is the drug Kymriah (tisagenlecleucel), which entered the market in October 2017. A novel gene- and cell-based immunotherapy, Kymriah was approved under FDA expedited pathways as a treatment for children and young adults who have relapsed or refractory

B-cell precursor acute lymphoblastic leukemia (ALL), a cancer that mainly affects the bone marrow and the blood.[31] According to some estimates, about 600 children and young adults per year will need the treatment. These cancer patients—as well as the general public—experienced sticker shock when the price for a one-time infusion of the drug was set by Novartis, the product developer, at $475,000. Yet additional costs, such as posttreatment bone-marrow transplantation, can run into the hundreds of thousands of dollars. Leonard Saltz, chief of gastrointestinal oncology at Memorial Sloan Kettering points out that immunotherapies like Kymriah "lead to a cascade of costs, propelled by serious side effects that require sophisticated management . . . For this class of drugs . . . consumers should think of the $475,000 as parts, not labor."[32]

Answering the question *should* public and private insurers pay for medical technologies that harm patients, that have an incomplete evidence base, that don't work, or that don't work any better than less expensive technologies— requires looking at the evidence of safety and effectiveness and deciding whether the evidence base justifies payer coverage. But that question raises additional questions: how much are we willing to pay for certain health outcomes, and does it matter who the patients are who need the drug?

In the case of Sovaldi and Harvoni, the two drugs can eliminate the virus for most patients, prevent the progression of hepatitis C to advanced liver disease, and possibly the need for a liver transplant. Following the logic adopted by many pharmaceutical companies that produce high-priced drugs, the manufacturer of Sovaldi and Harvoni argued that these drugs are actually much less expensive than alternative treatments for the liver disease caused by the virus. In contrast, insurance companies and some Medicaid directors pointed out that most people do not develop advanced liver disease, so this "savings" would not occur for people infected with the virus who do not develop clinical symptoms. The response by the payers ignores the public health perspective, however, because people who are infected but asymptomatic can infect other people. None of these arguments deals with two fundamental issues at play in the case of hepatitis C and many other debates about expensive treatments.

The first issue is price regulation. The debate about whether to cover the new hepatitis C drugs is shaped, in several ways, by the high cost of drugs, devices, and health care services in the United States. It is unlikely that Medicaid programs, prison health systems, and commercial health insurance companies would have placed restrictions on the use of these drugs if they were not so expensive. Similarly, the argument that these drugs are relatively inexpensive compared with alternative treatments ignores the possibility that the price of these other treatments is also unjustifiably high. The fact that a $1,000-per-day pill is less expensive than a combination of pills, surgeries, and other procedures that have prices neither the government nor private payers have negotiated effectively is not convincing. Debates that bring in evidence to justify the value of a particular medical care technology have to be placed in the context of the larger debate about how to set the price of these goods. This depends on political questions about how much, as a society, we are willing to spend on health care compared with other goods—and the degree to which we are willing to use the power of government to regulate the market. As with the other choices we describe, it is impossible and unwise to treat the answers to these questions as technical exercises that should be separated from "politics." We may not want decisions about drug regulation and drug prices to be driven by short-term electoral concerns or influenced by campaign contributions, but that does not help us get around the fact that choices of this sort do and must involve politics. Furthermore, they should be political because they involve choices about the nature of the society in which we live.

Second, the public and policy reactions to high spending on treatments is driven, at least in part, by perceptions of the groups in need of help. Media reports—including television ads from the companies marketing hepatitis C treatments—depict healthy-looking baby boomers as individuals who don't know they are infected with the virus or who have already been diagnosed with the disease. Yet those at high risk of getting hepatitis C are not typical baby boomers but injection drug users. Moreover, the rate of infection among prisoners is 30 times higher than in the general population, and the rate of infection is slightly higher in patients who receive Medicaid than those who are privately insured.[33]

Contrast the profile of the typical hepatitis C patient who will likely need public insurance coverage for access to Harvoni, with children who have muscular dystrophy and need Exondys 51, or with children and adolescents with cancer who need Kymriah. When considering the value of a medical technology in relation to the evidence of safety and effectiveness and its cost, emotional and thorny issues about who needs the drug are difficult to ignore. With regard to Kymriah, Dr. Michelle Hermiston, director of pediatric immunotherapy at UCSF Benioff Children's Hospital had this to say: "A kid's life is priceless . . . Any given kid has the potential to make financial impacts over a lifetime that far outweigh the costs of their cure. From this perspective, every child, in my mind, deserves the best curative therapy we can offer."[34] But Dr. Vinay Prasad, a hematologist-oncologist and assistant professor of medicine at the Oregon Health and Sciences University, noted that approximately 36 percent of patients who go into remission using Kymriah relapse within one year.[35] And Leonard Saltz asks, "If you've paid half a million dollars for drugs and half a million dollars for care, and a year later your cancer is back, is that a good deal?"[36]

Importantly, some payers are beginning to use novel coverage approaches. The CED coverage pathway under which CMS is paying for conditional access to amyloid PET imaging is one example. Whether and the extent to which private payers use CED is unknown. A disadvantage of this "outcomes-based" coverage approach is that insurers are subsidizing the research to obtain evidence of effectiveness. However, an advantage is that insurers are paying for a narrowly defined population of patients to get access to an intervention for a specific period of time, not for all patients diagnosed with the relevant condition to get it indefinitely in the clinical setting. If outcomes data of interest from a CED study do not meet the requisite evidentiary standards, the insurer is not required to expand coverage to all relevant patients in the clinical setting. Another example of an outcomes-based coverage approach is what Novartis agreed to for CMS coverage of Kymriah: the agency will only be required to pay for the drug if patients go into remission within one month of treatment.[37] Novartis reportedly is also offering this payment approach to private insurers.[38]

Whether public and private insurers will pay for medical technologies the FDA approves on the basis of RWE rather than data from RCTs or with limited data from RCTs remains to be seen. Steve Miller, the chief medical officer of Express Scripts, one of the nation's largest pharmacy benefits manager, points out that especially for drug approvals, "there is a lot of skepticism about using less than the most rigorous randomized trials to obtain evidence of safety and effectiveness." A key challenge, he said, is the lack of standards for evaluating RWE.[39] And Mike Kolodziej, a former Aetna national medical director for oncology strategies, notes that "Payers have to be convinced that the data is accurate and that the population in whom the data exists is representative of the membership of their beneficiaries . . . They don't want ineffective therapies that are toxic and expensive to be given in the rotation."[40]

Final Reflections

From one perspective, this book is about a bunch of wonky, scientific cases focused on particular diseases and particular medical technologies. But we believe that an examination of these cases offers a window into much larger disagreements in society about how to make collective decisions and how to set priorities. In documenting the choices that have to be made over a medical technology, we want to emphasize that these are not purely scientific matters and never will be. They involve debates about the goals of society and how we define what is fair. These decisions also have major consequences for the economy, for the size and shape of government, the distribution of power, and the allocation of resources. It is absurd to imagine that we can make decisions of this sort by getting rid of or getting around politics. Choices of this sort are what politics is about.

Clarifying the nature of these choices, raising questions about the evidence and arguments used to justify competing options, will help policy-makers muddle through the difficult choices. But beyond working to clarify the nature of these choices, we believe several interrelated and coordinated efforts are needed for (1) increasing public engagement in debates about evidentiary standards for medical technologies that is broader than the current patient advocacy model;[41] (2) providing public access to accurate, meaningful, and timely information from the FDA about the safety and effectiveness of medical technologies approved through the agency's expedited pathways, especially when approved on the basis of data from few clinical trials and sources other than RCTS; and (3) facilitating transparency about public and private payer coverage decision making.[42]

Public Engagement

As one of the leading proponents of public engagement in environmental policymaking put it, "the case for participation should begin with a normative argument—that a purely technocratic orientation is incompatible with democratic ideals."[43] The National Research Council echoed this view in 2008, saying, "public participation is intrinsic to democratic governance."[44] When individual patients and patient advocacy organizations testify at congressional and FDA hearings or submit written comments to regulatory agencies about proposed approval, withdrawal, or coverage decisions, they are involved in a form of public engagement. However, given the technical and moral complexities associated with decisions about medical technologies, we believe it is critical for broader public engagement regarding the standards and processes for health technology assessment and for patient access to medical technologies.

Justifications for broad public engagement in policymaking include the potential for (1) increasing the public's understanding about the values and interests at play in making difficult policy choices, (2) providing policymakers with multiple and diverse views about the goals of health technology assessment and of medical care, and (3) enhancing the legitimacy of policymaking processes and difficult policy choices. When discussing the value of medical technologies, the public should have an opportunity to set aside fears about "rationing," and policymakers should be encouraged to think carefully about the public's deeply held—even if poorly understood—values.[45] For example, policy analysis techniques like cost-benefit analysis tend to exclude some values that cannot easily be quantified.[46]

Public engagement beyond agency hearings and notice and comment periods for proposed regulatory action include town hall meetings, citizens' juries, public surveys, deliberative polling, and referendums.[47] Some forms of public engagement, such as citizens' juries, are specifically designed as deliberative activities rather than activities for providing policymakers with information about public perspectives.[48] Public deliberation is typically considered useful and appropriate for addressing policy problems that involve high levels of value conflict and for which technical expertise is insufficient or where the institutions charged with making decisions are not trusted.[49] Disputes about medical technologies are well suited to public deliberation. Yet there are many challenges to carrying out public engagement activities—especially those involving deliberative approaches: Who should carry out deliberative activities? Who should be included in such activities? When should a deliberative activity occur, and how should the topics for discussion be selected? The literature on deliberation suggests broad criteria for conducting successful and legitimate deliberation, though not all of the questions posed here have been adequately addressed by proponents of deliberation.

Evidence from public engagement efforts in other countries suggests that processes can be developed to meet some of the challenges. During the past decade, Canada has employed a citizens' jury approach to get public input about priority-setting criteria[50] and about the evidence thresholds that should be used for funding new medical technologies.[51] In the UK, the National Institute for Health and Care Excellence (NICE) appraises new drugs and new indications for existing, licensed medications, along with other technologies (such as medical devices), surgical and diagnostic procedures, and public health interventions. NICE derives conclusions about whether treatments or interventions are therapeutically beneficial and cost-effective, as compared to other relevant alternatives, by reviewing a range of available evidence, most often assembled and synthesized by a publicly funded network of academic institutions.

Recommendations for technologies that the UK's National Health Service should adopt are based on a number of considerations, namely comparative clinical and cost-effectiveness, disease burden, and social values. Most of the attention is focused on NICE's cost-effectiveness analysis, in which it makes judgments about value for money, usually based on an informal threshold range of £20,000 to £30,000 per QALY (quality-adjusted life year). But to identify appropriate social values in the appraisal process, NICE also conducts deliberations among members of the public. In 2002 NICE established the Citizens Council to ensure the perspective of the public is reflected in the methodology and processes that NICE uses to develop its guidance. The Citizens Council is a panel of 30 members of the public that largely reflect the demographic characteristics of the UK. They address the moral and ethical issues that NICE should consider when making recommendations about the use of medical technologies.[52]

Will the U.S. political system allow anything that looks like the examples from Canada and the United Kingdom to work here? We are not hopeful that this is likely in the near term at the national level. PCORI is supposed to be "patient centered," and its operations are influenced by the community-based participatory research movement, in which the general public is given an opportunity to shape the questions researchers address, the interpretation of evidence, and the recommendations that flow from study findings. At the same time, PCORI is banned by Congress from considering certain questions and is not allowed to consider the type of incremental cost-effectiveness analysis used by other countries and private payers in the United States. Although PCORI may consider costs, in practice they shy away from this as well because leaders of the agency are fearful that members of Congress may attack it if they do so. These fears are well founded, since Congress has already proposed eliminating the agency.

As an organization whose task is to make evidence-based recommendations about preventive services and technologies, the USPSTF is composed of 16 volunteer members who are nationally recognized experts in prevention, evidence-based medicine, and primary care. In response to complaints about the lack of transparency and opportunity for public input, in 2011 the organization began inviting the public to comment on its draft research plans, and in 2013 to comment on its draft evidence reviews.[53] However, it is unclear from the USPSTF Web site whether public comments are submitted and by whom.

The FDA has initiated several patient engagement initiatives, most recently in response to requirements of the Cures Act. In 2015 the agency helped fund a project under the auspices of the Medical Device Innovation Consortium to develop a framework for incorporating patient preference information into the agency's regulatory benefit-risk assessments of medical technologies.[54] Importantly, the report from this project emphasizes that "[p]atient preference information can be a supplement to clinical and safety data and provide additional information for consideration by the FDA but does not change the existing regulatory requirements."[55] In September 2015, the agency announced in the *Federal Register* that it was establishing a Patient Engagement Advisory Committee to provide advice to the FDA "on complex issues relating to medical devices, regulation of devices, and their use by patients."[56] Topics the committee may consider include FDA "guidance and policies, clinical trial or registry design, patient preference study design, benefit risk determinations, device labeling, unmet clinical needs, available alternatives, patient reported outcomes and device-related quality of life or health status issues, and other patient-related topics."[57]

In the Cures Act, Congress specifically mandated that the FDA develop guidance "regarding the collection of patient experience data, and the use of such data and related information in drug development."[58] The FDA held its first public workshop on patient-focused drug development in December 2017 to discuss "methodological approaches that a person seeking to collect patient experience data for submission to FDA to inform regulatory decision-making may use."[59] Prior to the workshop, the agency released a discussion document that provided the basis for informing the development of the

Cures-mandated guidance documents that will be designed to "facilitate col-lection and submission of usable patient experience data for medical product development and regulatory decision-making."[60]

The FDA's patient engagement initiatives are important steps toward giv-ing patients a voice in the regulatory process governing the development and assessment of drugs and devices. But these initiatives do not answer ques-tions about how much influence certain voices should have or whether all voices—including those that conflict with patients' urgency narratives—will be welcome and heard.[61] Moreover, the FDA's engagement approaches do not include processes for broad public deliberation about the complex values that are at play in developing, raising, or lowering evidentiary standards regarding the safety and effectiveness of medical technologies.

Access to Postapproval Data

Over the past decade, the FDA has improved reporting through its publicly accessible Web site of safety alerts, adverse event reports, recalls, and market withdrawals for drugs; recalls for biologics; and recalls and safety communi-cations regarding medical devices. On January 16, 2018, the agency announced a new pilot initiative to enhance transparency of clinical trial information.[62] The FDA will invite product developers to voluntarily participate in the pilot project, with the goal of obtaining nine new drug applications that involve novel products and specific scientific questions of interest. After a drug has been approved, the FDA will post on its Web site parts of the clinical study reports that the product developers submitted to the FDA supporting their application for market approval. The agency will provide the body of the study report, the study's protocol and amendments, and the statistical analysis plan that was used for each of the pivotal studies. The purpose of making this information publicly available, said the FDA, is to "provide stakeholders with more information on the clinical evidence supporting a drug application and more transparency in the FDA's decision-making process."[63]

At this time, for the drugs and biologics that received accelerated approval on condition of postapproval requirements, it is difficult to track which prod-ucts have such requirements and whether those requirements were met. It is too soon to know whether the pilot transparency initiative will improve pub-lic access to information about mandated postapproval studies. So that patients receive safe and effective therapeutic drugs, it is essential that the public have access to accurate, meaningful, and timely information from the FDA about information from postapproval studies, especially when the prod-uct entered the market on the basis of data from few clinical trials, from sources other than RCTs, and from surrogate end points. Providing such information is not only critical to protect the public's health but for maintaining the FDA's reputation and legitimacy in regulating access to safe and effective medical technologies.[64]

Public and Private Payer Transparency

Although CMS posts on its Web site the coverage decisions made under the NCD and CED pathways, many stakeholders complain that the agency is not as transparent as it could be about how it weighs evidence of safety and effectiveness of technologies and decides which outcomes take precedence over others. And as the Office of Inspector General pointed out, there is little transparency about the decision-making process for the vast majority of coverage decisions made through the LCD process.[65] Even less is known about coverage criteria and decision making of state Medicaid agencies and private payers. Interviews with a small sample of private payers regarding the *Oncotype* DX gene expression profiling test for breast cancer recurrence indicate that some payers preferred to make a coverage decision based on health outcomes evidence regarding impact on patient disease and survival, though others were willing to define clinical utility as evidence that test information affected clinical decision making.[66] Other studies of private-payer coverage for genetic testing indicate that some payers define clinical utility as evidence that the genetic test information affects clinical decisions, while other payers define clinical utility more narrowly, requiring evidence from RCTs about clinical outcomes of patients who underwent testing.[67]

Federal government policymakers could require greater transparency at CMS and by state Medicaid programs, though given the political battle in the early days of the Medicare program to establish coverage criteria, fostering greater transparency will be no easy task. And private payers are notoriously unwilling to reveal details of the criteria upon which they make coverage decisions. However, as new drugs and biologics become available—particularly treatments for seriously ill and dying patients—private insurers may need to be more transparent—and might even consider engaging with the public to open the discussion about assessing the value of medical technologies for the purpose of payer coverage.

Looking Forward

Disputes about evidentiary standards for technology assessment are never definitely resolved. Rather, they evolve over time and carry with them shifting alliances across stakeholder groups, policy framing and reframing, and negotiated policy responses to values and interests foregrounded at differing points in time. The cases in this book provide windows into how values and interests shape the way evidence is defined, gathered, and evaluated, as well as how the fluidity of those values and interests play out in relation to the type of technology at issue, the setting in which it is evaluated, and the complex issues associated with its value and cost. Such information may provide a more accurate lens through which to identify the forces that account for ongoing and seemingly intractable disputes about assessing a medical technology's value for diagnosing, preventing, or treating diseases and disorders. Studies such as this one that bring clarity to complex issues can contribute to the public dialogue at a time when clarity is often lacking.

Notes

Chapter 1

1. Marcel Proust, *Swann's Way* (Mineola, NY: Dover, 2002).

2. Institute of Medicine, *Evidence-Based Medicine and the Changing Nature of Healthcare: Meeting Summary* (Washington, D.C.: National Academies Press, 2008); Institute of Medicine, *Initial National Priorities for Comparative Effectiveness Research* (Washington, D.C.: National Academies Press, 2009); R. Platt, N. E. Kass, and D. McGraw, "Ethics, Regulation, and Comparative Effectiveness Research. Time for Change," *Journal of the American Medical Association* 311, no. 15 (2014): 1497–98; Miriam Solomon, *Making Medical Knowledge* (Oxford: Oxford University Press, 2015); C. Sorenson, M. K. Gusmano, and A. Oliver, "The Politics of Comparative Effectiveness Research: Lessons from Recent History," *Journal of Health Politics, Policy and Law* 3, no. 1 (2014): 139–69, at 40; John Wennberg, "Forty Years of Unwarranted Variation—And Still Counting," *Health Policy* 114 (2014): 1–2.

3. Sorenson, Gusmano, and Oliver, "The Politics of Comparative Effectiveness Research: Lessons from Recent History."

4. Richard A. Rettig, et al., *False Hope: Bone Marrow Transplantation for Breast Cancer* (New York: Oxford University Press, 2007); Katherine Cooper Wulff, Franklin G. Miller, and Steven D. Pearson, "Can Coverage Be Rescinded When Negative Trial Results Threaten a Popular Procedure? The Ongoing Saga of Vertebroplasty," *Health Affairs* 30, no. 12 (2011): 2269–76.

5. Daniel Carpenter, *Reputation and Power: Organizational Image and Pharmaceutical Regulation at the FDA* (Princeton, NJ: Princeton University Press, 2014); Alex Faulkner, *Medical Technology into Healthcare and Society* (London: Palgrave, 2009); Rettig, et al., *False Hope: Bone Marrow Transplantation for Breast Cancer.*

6. Richard E. Ashcroft, "Current Epistemological Problems in Evidence Based Medicine," *Journal of Medical Ethics* 30 (2004): 131–35; Solomon, *Making Medical Knowledge*; Stefan Timmermans and Marc Berg, *The Gold Standard: The Challenge of Evidence-Based Medicine and Standardization in Health Care* (Philadelphia: Temple University Press, 2010); Sandra J. Tannenbaum, "Particularism in Health Care: Challenging the Authority of the Aggregate," *Journal of Evaluation in Clinical Practice* 20 (2014): 934–41.

7. John Abraham and Rachel Ballinger, "The Neoliberal Regulatory State, Industry Interests, and the Ideological Penetration of Scientific Knowledge: Deconstructing the Redefinition of Carcinogens in Pharmaceuticals," *Science, Technology & Human Values* 37, no. 5 (2012): 443–77; Carpenter, *Reputation and Power: Organizational Image and Pharmaceutical Regulation at the FDA*; Faulkner, *Medical Technology into Healthcare and Society*; Rettig, et al., *False Hope: Bone Marrow Transplantation for Breast Cancer*.

8. Daniel Béland, "Ideas and Social Policy: An Institutionalist Perspective," *Social Policy & Administration* 39, no. 1 (2005): 1–18; John L. Campbell, "Ideas, Politics and Public Policy," *Annual Review of Sociology* 28 (2002): 21–38; Peter A. Hall, "The Role of Interests, Institutions and Ideas in the Comparative Political Economy of the Industrialized Nations," in *Comparative Politics: Rationality, Culture, and Structure*, eds. Mark Irving Lichbach and Alan S. Zuckerman (New York: Cambridge University Press, 1997), 174–207; Ellen M. Immergut, *Health Politics: Interests and Institutions in Western Europe* (Cambridge: CUP Archive, 1992); Theodore Marmor, Richard Freeman, and Kieke Okma, "Comparative Perspectives and Policy Learning in the World of Health Care," *Journal of Comparative Policy* 7, no. 4 (2005): 331–48.

9. National Geographic, "The War on Science," February 17, 2015, http://ngm.nationalgeographic.com/2015/03/science-doubters/achenbach-text.

10. Michael Siegel, "Don't Let Alternative Facts Deter Congress from Fixing e-Cigarette Regulations," *Washington Examiner*, May 2, 2017, http://www.washingtonexaminer.com/dont-let-alternative-facts-deter-congress-from-fixing-e-cigarette-regulations/article/262182.

11. Jonathan J. Darrow, Jerry Avorn, and Aaron S. Kesselheim, "New FDA Breakthrough-Drug Category—Implications for Patients," *New England Journal of Medicine* 370, no. 13 (2014): 1252–58; Vinay Prasad and Sham Mailankody, "The Accelerated Approval of Oncologic Drugs: Lessons from Ponatinib," *Journal of the American Medical Association* 311, no. 4 (2014): 353–54; Rettig, et al., *False Hope: Bone Marrow Transplantation for Breast Cancer*.

12. Ashcroft, "Current Epistemological Problems in Evidence Based Medicine"; Faulkner, *Medical Technology into Healthcare and Society*; Trisha Greenhalgh, Jeremy Howick, and Neal Naskrey, for the Evidence Based Medicine Renaissance Group, "Evidence Based Medicine: A Movement in Crisis?" *BMJ* (2014): 348, g3725; Rettig, et al., *False Hope: Bone Marrow Transplantation for Breast Cancer*; Solomon, *Making Medical Knowledge*; Tannenbaum, "Particularism in Health Care: Challenging the Authority of the Aggregate"; Timmermans and Berg, *The Gold Standard: The Challenge of Evidence-Based Medicine and Standardization in Health Care*.

13. Michael K. Gusmano and Gregory E. Kaebnick, "Clarifying the Role of Values in Cost-Effectiveness," *Health Economics, Policy and Law* 11, no. 4 (2016): 439–43.

14. Stanley Kelley, *Professional Public Relations and Political Power* (Baltimore, MD: Johns Hopkins University Press, 1956).

15. Edmund F. Wehrle, "For a Healthy America," *Labor's Heritage* 28 (Summer 1993): 40.

16. Kelley, *Professional Public Relations and Political Power.*

17. David Williams, "ObamaCare Demonstrates Dangers of Government Interference," *The Hill*, November 2, 2016, http://origin-nyi.thehill.com/blogs /pundits-blog/healthcare/304066-obamacare-demonstrates-dangers-of -government-interference.

18. Andrew von Eschenbach, "Medical Innovation: How the U.S. Can Retain Its Lead," *Wall Street Journal*, February 14, 2012, https://www.wsj.com/articles /SB10001424052970203646004577215403399350874.

19. Paul Howard, "To Lower Drug Prices, Innovate, Don't Regulate," *New York Times*, September 23, 2015, https://www.nytimes.com/roomfordebate/2015/09 /23/should-the-government-impose-drug-price-controls/to-lower-drug-prices -innovate-dont-regulate.

20. Peter Arno and Michael H. Davis, "At Issue: Should Medicare Be Allowed to Negotiate Drug Prices?" *CQ Researcher* 26, no. 20 (2016): 473.

21. Solomon, *Making Medical Knowledge.*

22. Uwe Reinhardt, "Divide et Impera: Protecting the Growth of Health Care Incomes (COSTS)," *Health Economics* 21 (2012): 41–54.

23. Liyan Chen, "The Most Profitable Industries in 2016," *Forbes*, December 21, 2016, https://www.forbes.com/sites/liyanchen/2015/12/21/the-most-profitable -industries-in-2016/#1e6b80ab5716.

24. Tiffany C. Wright, "The Average Profit Margin of Pharmaceuticals," *azcentral.com*, https://yourbusiness.azcentral.com/average-profit-marginphar -maceuticals-20671.html.

25. U.S. Government Accountability Office, "Medical Device Companies: Trends in Reported Net Sales and Profits Before and After Implementation of the Patient Protection and Affordable Care Act," June 30, 2015, https://www.gao.gov /products/GAO-15-635R.

26. David Truman, *The Government Process: Political Interests and Public Opinion* (New York: Alfred A. Knopf, 1951).

27. Carpenter, *Reputation and Power: Organizational Image and Pharmaceutical Regulation at the FDA*; Stephen Epstein, *AIDS, Activism and the Politics of Knowledge* (Berkeley: University of California Press, 1996); Faulkner, *Medical Technology into Healthcare and Society*; Rettig, et al., *False Hope: Bone Marrow Transplantation for Breast Cancer.*

28. Jerry Avorn and Aaron S. Kesselheim, "The 21st Century Cures Act—Will It Take Us Back in Time?" *New England Journal of Medicine* 372, no. 26 (2015): 2473–75; Insoo Hyun, "Allowing Innovative Stem Cell-Based Therapies Outside of Clinical Trials: Ethical and Policy Challenges," *Journal of Law, Medicine & Ethics* 38, no. 2 (2010): 277–85; Olle Lindvall and Insoo Hyun, "Medical Innovation versus Stem Cell Tourism," *Science* 324, no. 5935 (2009): 1664–65.

29. Avorn and Kesselheim, "The 21st Century Cures Act—Will It Take Us Back in Time?"; Hyun, "Allowing Innovative Stem Cell-Based Therapies Outside of Clinical Trials: Ethical and Policy Challenges"; Lindvall and Hyun, "Medical Innovation versus Stem Cell Tourism."

30. 21st Century Cures Act, Public Law 114-255, December 13, 2016.

31. Katie Thomas, "Trump Vows to Ease Rules for Drug Makers, but Again Zeros in on Prices," *New York Times*, January 31, 2017, https://www.nytimes.com/2017/01/31/health/trump-vows-to-ease-rules-for-drug-makers-but-prices-remain-a-focus.html.

32. Seth D. Ginsberg, "What to Do If You're Denied Coverage for a New Cholesterol Drug You Need," *U.S. News and World Report*, September 9, 2016, http://health.usnews.com/health-news/patient-advice/articles/2016-09-09/what-to-do-if-youre-denied-coverage-for-a-new-cholesterol-drug-you-need.

33. Robert Handfield and Josh Feldstein, "Insurance Companies' Perspectives on the Orphan Drug Pipeline," *American Health & Drug Benefits* 6, no. 9 (2013): 589–98.

34. Susan Bartlett Foote, "Why Medicare Cannot Promulgate a National Coverage Rule: A Case of Regula Mortis," *Journal of Health Politics, Policy and Law* 27, no. 5 (2002): 707–30; Muriel R. Gillick, "Medicare Coverage for Technological Innovations—Time for New Criteria?" *New England Journal of Medicine* 350, no. 21 (2004): 2199–201; Muriel R. Gillick, "The Technological Imperative and the Battle for the Hearts of America," *Perspectives in Biology and Medicine* 50, no. 2 (2007): 276–94; Rettig, et al., *False Hope: Bone Marrow Transplantation for Breast Cancer*; Wulff, Miller, and Pearson, "Can Coverage Be Rescinded When Negative Trial Results Threaten a Popular Procedure? The Ongoing Saga of Vertebroplasty."

35. M. A. Jogerst, *Reform in the House of Commons: The Select Committee System* (Lexington: University of Kentucky Press, 1993).

36. Peter A. Hall, "Policy Paradigms, Social Learning, and the State: The Case of Economic Policymaking in Britain," *Comparative Politics* 25, no. 3 (1993): 275–96; Jogerst, *Reform in the House of Commons: The Select Committee System*; Paul Pierson, "When Effect Becomes Cause: Policy Feedback and Political Change," *World Politics* 45, no. 4 (1993): 595–628.

37. Hall, "Policy Paradigms, Social Learning, and the State: The Case of Economic Policymaking in Britain"; Hugh Heclo, *Modern Social Politics in Britain and Sweden: From Relief to Income Maintenance* (New Haven, CT: Yale University Press, 1987); Jogerst, *Reform in the House of Commons: The Select Committee System*; Theda Skocpol, *Protecting Soldiers and Mothers: The Political Origins of Social Policy in the United States* (Cambridge, MA: Belknap Press of Harvard University Press, 1992); Margert Weir, Ann Shola Orloff, and Theda Skocpol, *The Politics of Social Policy in the United States* (Princeton, NJ: Princeton University Press, 1988).

38. Hall, "Policy Paradigms, Social Learning, and the State: The Case of Economic Policymaking in Britain."

39. Mary Ann Chirba and Alice A. Noble, "Our Bodies, Our Cells: FDA Regulation of Autologous Adult Stem Cell Therapies," *Bill of Health Blog*, June 2, 2013, http://blogs.harvard.edu/billofhealth/2013/06/02/our-bodies-our-cells-fda-regulation-of-autologous-adult-stem-cell-therapies/; Karen J. Maschke and Michael K. Gusmano, "Evidence and Access to Biomedical Interventions: The Case of Stem Cell Treatments," *Journal of Health Politics, Policy and Law* 41, no. 5 (2016): 917–36.

40. Margaret L. Eaton and Donald Kennedy, *Innovation in Medical Technology: Ethical Issues and Challenges* (Baltimore: Johns Hopkins University Press, 2007); Lindvall and Hyun, "Medical Innovation versus Stem Cell Tourism."

41. Solomon, *Making Medical Knowledge*; Tannenbaum, "Particularism in Health Care: Challenging the Authority of the Aggregate"; Timmermans and Berg, *The Gold Standard: The Challenge of Evidence-Based Medicine and Standardization in Health Care.*

42. Faulkner, *Medical Technology into Healthcare and Society*; Rettig, et al., *False Hope: Bone Marrow Transplantation for Breast Cancer.*

43. Robert M. Ball, "What Medicare's Architects Had in Mind," *Health Affairs* 14, no. 4 (1995): 62–72; Theodore Marmor, *The Politics of Medicare* (Chicago: Aldine, 1973).

44. Institute of Medicine, *Medicare: A Strategy for Quality Assurance, Volume I.* (Washington, D.C.: National Academy Press, 1990).

45. Marilyn Moon, *Medicare Now and in the Future* (Washington, D.C.: Urban Institute Press, 1993).

46. Title XVIII of the Social Security Act.

47. Ball, "What Medicare's Architects Had in Mind."

48. A. Donabedian, "Evaluating the Quality of Medical Care," *Milbank Memorial Fund Quarterly* 44, no. 3, pt. 2 (1966): 166–203.

49. David Blumenthal and Charles M. Kilo, "A Report Card on Continuous Quality Improvement," *Milbank Quarterly* 76, no. 4 (1998): 625–48; J. M. Juran, *A History of Managing for Quality* (Milwaukee: ASQC Quality Press, 1995); W. A. Shewhart, *Statistical Method from the Viewpoint of Quality Control* (Mineola, NY: Dover, 1986).

50. Marmor, *The Politics of Medicare.*

51. Michael K. Gusmano, "Health Systems Performance and the Politics of Cancer Survival," *World Medical and Health Policy* 5, no. 1 (2013): 76–84; Wendell Potter, "Does the U.S. Have the World's Best Health Care System? Yes, if You're Talking about the Third World," *Huffington Post*, November 28, 2011, https://www.huffingtonpost.com/wendell-potter/does-the-us-have-the-best_b_1116105.html.

52. Kevin Boland, "CBO Confirms ObamaCare Will Increase Prescription Drug Prices," Speaker Paul Ryan (website), November 4, 2010, https://www.speaker.gov/general/cbo-confirms-obamacare-will-increase-prescription-drug-prices.

53. Michelle Moons, "Mike Pence: 'We Need Every Republican in Congress,' Every American for Healthcare 'Battle,'" *Breitbart News*, March 11, 2017, http://www.breitbart.com/big-government/2017/03/11/pence-need-every-republican-congress-every-american-healthcare-battle/.

Chapter 2

1. Reed Tuckson and Daniel S. Blumenthal, "Why Aren't Millions of Americans Getting Preventive Care?" STAT, April 15, 2016, https://www.statnews.com/2016/04/15/preventive-care-public-health/.

2. Martin A. Makary and Michael Daniel, "Medical Error—The Third Leading Cause of Death in the U.S.," *BMJ* May 2016; 353: i2139. doi: 10.1136/bmj.i2139.

3. David M. Cutler, *Your Money or Your Life: Strong Medicine for America's Health Care System* (New York: Oxford University Press, 2004).

4. Ajay E. Kuriyan, et al., "Vision Loss after Intravitreal Injection of Autologous 'Stem Cells' for AMD," *New England Journal of Medicine* 376, no. 11 (2017): 1047–53; Laurie McGinley, "FDA Cracks Down on Stem-Cell Clinics, Including One Using Smallpox Vaccine in Cancer Patients," *Washington Post*, August 28, 2017, https://www.washingtonpost.com/news/to-your-health/wp/2017/08/28/fda-cracks-down-on-stem-cell-clinics-including-one-using-smallpox-vaccine-in-cancer-patients/?utm_term=.67b4aa33d45d&wpisrc=al_alert-hse&wpmk=1.

5. Robert M. Ball, "What Medicare's Architects Had in Mind," *Health Affairs* 14, no. 4 (1995): 62–72.

6. Institute of Medicine, *Medicare: A Strategy for Quality Assurance, Volume I* (Washington, D.C.: National Academies Press, 1990).

7. Marilyn Moon, *Medicare Now and in the Future* (Washington, D.C.: The Urban Institute Press, 1993).

8. Ibid.

9. Michael K. Gusmano, "Health Systems Performance and the Politics of Cancer Survival," *World Medical & Health Policy* 5, no. 1 (2013): 76–84.

10. Robert M. Ball, "What Medicare's Architects Had in Mind."

11. Avedis Donabedian, "Evaluating the Quality of Medical Care," *The Milbank Memorial Fund Quarterly* 44, no. 3, pt. 2 (1966): 166–203.

12. David Blumenthal and Charles M. Kilo, "A Report Card on Continuous Quality Improvement," *The Milbank Quarterly* 76, no. 4 (2001): 625–48.

13. Laura E. Bothwell, Jeremy A. Greene, Scott H. Podolsky, and David S. Jones, "Assessing the Gold Standard—Lessons from the History of RCTs," *New England Journal of Medicine* 374 (2016): 2175–81.

14. Harry M. Marks, *The Progress of Experiment: Science and Therapeutic Reform in the United States, 1900–1990* (Cambridge: Cambridge University Press, 2000).

15. Miriam Solomon, *Making Medical Knowledge* (Oxford: Oxford University Press, 2015).

16. Julius M. Cruse, "History of Medicine: The Metamorphosis of Scientific Medicine in the Ever-Present Past," *American Journal of the Medical Sciences* 318, no. 3 (1999): 171–80.

17. Abraham Flexner, "Medical Education in the United States and Canada. A Report to the Carnegie Foundation for the Advancement of Teaching," 1910, http://archive.carnegiefoundation.org/pdfs/elibrary/Carnegie_Flexner_Report.pdf.

18. Molly Cooke, et al., "American Medical Education 100 Years after the Flexner Report," *New England Journal of Medicine* 355, no. 13 (2006): 1339–44.

19. Roger L. Sur and Philipp Dahm, "History of Evidence-Based Medicine," *Indian Journal of Urology* 27, no. 4 (2011): 487–89.

20. Daniel Carpenter, *Reputation and Power: Organizational Image and Pharmaceutical Regulation at the FDA* (Princeton, NJ: Princeton University Press, 2014); Alex Faulkner, *Medical Technology into Healthcare and Society* (London: Palgrave, 2009).

21. James Morone, *The Democratic Wish: Popular Participation and the Limits of American Democracy* (New York: Basic Books, 1990), 266.

22. Paul Starr, *The Social Transformation of American Medicine: The Rise of a Sovereign Profession and the Making of a Vast Industry* (New York: Basic Books, 1982).

23. Theodor J. Litman and Leonard S. Robins, *Health Politics and Policy,* Second Edition (New York: Delmar Series in Health Services Administration, 1991), 273–74.

24. Michael K. Gusmano and Daniel Callahan, "Value for Money: Use with Care," *Annals of Internal Medicine* 154, no. 3 (2011): 207–08.

25. Starr, *The Social Transformation of American Medicine: The Rise of a Sovereign Profession and the Making of a Vast Industry,* 408.

26. Ibid.

27. Ibid., 409; Aaron Wildavsky, "Doing Better and Feeling Worse: The Political Pathology of Health Policy," in *The Art and Craft of Policy Analysis,* ed. Aaron Wildavsky (London: Palgrave Macmillan, 1979), 284–308; Ivan Illich, *Medical Nemesis: The Expropriation of Health* (London: Calder & Boyars, 1974).

28. Daniel Callahan, *What Kind of Life: The Limits of Medical Progress* (New York: Simon and Schuster, 1990).

29. Lisa F. Berkman, Ichiro Kawachi, and Maria Glymour, eds., *Social Epidemiology,* Second Edition (Oxford: Oxford University Press, 2014); Richard Wilkinson and Michael Marmot, eds., *The Solid Facts,* Second Edition (Copenhagen: The World Health Organization, 2003).

30. Starr, *The Social Transformation of American Medicine: The Rise of a Sovereign Profession and the Making of a Vast Industry.*

31. Ibid.

32. Robert W. Fogel. "The Extension of Life in Developed Countries and Its Implications for Social Policy in the Twenty-First Century," *Population and Development Review* 26 (2000): 291–317.

33. Ibid., 310.

34. Gusmano and Callahan, "Value for Money: Use with Care."

35. Cutler, *Your Money or Your Life: Strong Medicine for America's Health Care System.*

36. K. L. White, T. Franklin Williams, and Bernard G. Greenberg. "The Ecology of Medical Care, 1961," *Bulletin of the New York Academy of Medicine* 73, no. 1 (1996): 187.

37. Edward Berkowitz, "History of Health Services Research Project Interview with Barbara Starfield," U.S. National Library of Medicine, August 8, 1998, https://www.nlm.nih.gov/hmd/nichsr/starfield.html.

38. Ibid.

39. John Wennberg and A. Gittelsohn, "Small Area Variations in Health Care Delivery: A Population-Based Health Information System Can Guide Planning and Regulatory Decision-Making," *Science* 182, no. 4117 (1973): 1102–08.

40. John Wennberg, "Forty Years of Unwarranted Variation—And Still Counting," *Health Policy* 114 (2014): 1–2.

41. R. H. Brook, K. N. Williams, and J. E. Rolph, "Controlling the Use and Cost of Medical Services: The New Mexico Experimental Medical Care Review Organization—A Four-Year Case Study," *Medical Care* 16, no. 9, Suppl. (1978): 1–76; Robert H. Brook, et al., "Geographic Variations in the Use of Services: Do They Have any Clinical Significance?" *Health Affairs* 3, no. 2 (1984): 63–73; Robert H. Brook, et al., "A Method for Detailed Assessment of the Appropriateness of Medical Technologies," *International Journal of Technology Assessment in Health Care* 2, no. 1 (1986): 53–63; Robert H. Brook, "Practice Guidelines and Practicing Medicine: Are They Compatible?" *Journal of the American Medical Association* 262 (1989): 3027–30.

42. Brook, et al., "Geographic Variations in the Use of Services: Do They Have any Clinical Significance?"

43. Cochrane United States, http://us.cochrane.org/; GRADE Working Group, http://www.gradeworkinggroup.org/; G. Guyatt, et al., "The Vexing Problem of Guidelines and Conflict of Interest: A Potential Solution," *Annals of Internal Medicine* 152, no. 11 (2010): 738–41.

44. Rosemary Stevens, *The Public-Private Health Care State: Essays on the History of American Health Care Policy* (New Brunswick, NJ: Transaction Publishers, 2007).

45. Bradford H. Gray, "The Legislative Battle Over Health Services Research," *Health Affairs* 11, no. 4 (1992): 38–66.

46. Bruce Allen Bimber, *The Politics of Expertise in Congress: The Rise and Fall of the Office of Technology Assessment* (Albany, NY: SUNY Press, 1996).

47. Dennis Cotter, "The National Center for Health Technology: Lessons Learned," *Health Affairs Blog*, January 22, 2009, https://www.healthaffairs.org/do/10.1377/hblog20090122.000490/full/.

48. C. Sorenson, M. K. Gusmano, and A. Oliver, "The Politics of Comparative Effectiveness Research: Lessons from Recent History," *Journal of Health Politics, Policy and Law* 3, no. 1 (2014): 139–169.

49. Ibid.

50. Gray, "The Legislative Battle Over Health Services Research."

51. John A. Wennberg, "AHCPR And the Strategy for Health Care Reform," *Health Affairs* 11, no. 4 (1992): 67–72.

52. Gray, "The Legislative Battle Over Health Services Research."

53. Ibid.

54. Bryan Luce and Rebecca Singer Cohen, "Health Technology Assessment in the United States," *International Journal of Technology Assessment in Health Care* 25, Suppl. 1 (2009): 33–41.

55. Gray, "The Legislative Battle Over Health Services Research."

56. Bradford H. Gray, Michael K. Gusmano, and Sara R. Collins, "AHCPR and the Politics of Health Services Research," *Health Affairs Web Exclusive*, June 25, 2003, https://s3.amazonaws.com/academia.edu.documents/39679961/AHCPR_and_the_Changing_Politics_of_Healt20151104-22646-1hdvtk4.pdf?AWSAccessKeyId=AKIAIWOWYYGZ2Y53UL3A&Expires=1516159851&Signature=wH9Ez2DgqwTmzAA1dwUOcivPiyE%3D&response-content-disposition=inline%3B%20filename%3DAHCPR_And_The_Changing_Politics_Of_Healt.pdf.

57. Sorenson, et al., "The Politics of Comparative Effectiveness Research: Lessons from Recent History."

58. J. M. Eisenberg and D. Zarin, "Health Technology Assessment in the United States. Past, Present, and Future," *International Journal of Technology Assessment in Health Care* 18, no. 2 (2002): 192–98.

59. Gray, et al., "AHCPR and the Politics of Health Services Research."

60. John E. Wennberg, "The More Things Change . . . The Federal Government's Role in Evaluative Sciences," *Health Affairs* 2003: W3-308–10.

61. Thomas A. Birkland, "Focusing Events, Mobilization, and Agenda Setting," *Journal of Public Policy* 18, no. 1 (1998): 53–74; Peter A. Hall and Rosemary C. R. Taylor, "Political Science and the Three New Institutionalisms," *Political Studies* 44, no 5 (1996): 936–57.

62. Institute of Medicine, *To Err Is Human: Building a Safer Health System* (Washington, D.C.: National Academies Press, 1999); Institute of Medicine. *Crossing the Quality Chasm: New Health System for the 21st Century* (Washington, D.C.: National Academies Press, 2001).

63. Donald Berwick, "A User's Manual for the IOM's 'Quality Chasm' Report," *Health Affairs* 21, no. 3 (2002): 80–90.

64. Bruce C. Vladeck and Thomas Rice, "Market Failure and the Failure of Discourse: Facing Up to the Power of Sellers," *Health Affairs* 28, no. 5 (2009): 1305–15.

65. Sorenson et al., "The Politics of Comparative Effectiveness Research: Lessons from Recent History."

66. Gail R. Wilensky, "Developing a Center for Comparative Effectiveness Information," *Health Affairs* 25, no. 6 (2006): w572–w585.

67. P. J. Neumann, A. B. Rosen, and M. C. Weinstein, "Medicare and Cost-Effectiveness Analysis," *New England Journal of Medicine* 353, no. 14 (2005): 1516–22.

68. Ibid.

69. John Reichard, "Baucus, Conrad Offer Bill Creating Comparative Effectiveness Institute," *Washington Health Policy Week in Review*, August 4, 2008, http://www.commonwealthfund.org/publications/newsletters/washington -health-policy-in-review/2008/aug/washington-health-policy-week-in-review -august-4-2008/baucus-conrad-offer-bill-creating-comparative-effectiveness -institute.

70. John K. Iglehart, "The Political Fight Over Comparative Effectiveness Research," *Health Affairs* 29, no. 10 (2010): 1757–60.

71. James D. Chambers, P. J. Neumann, and M. J. Buxton, "Does Medicare Have an Implicit Cost-Effectiveness Threshold?" *Medical Decision Making* 30, no. 4 (2010): E14–27.

72. Sorenson, et al., "The Politics of Comparative Effectiveness Research: Lessons from Recent History."

73. Iglehart, "The Political Fight Over Comparative Effectiveness Research."

74. National Pharmaceutical Council, "Health Affairs CER Briefing Highlights Key Issues," National Pharmaceutical Council Newsletter, October 2010,

http://www.npcnow.org/newsroom/commentary/health-affairs-cer-briefing
-highlights-key-issues.

75. Fred Schulte, "Is Obamacare's Research Institute Worth the Billions?" NPR, August 4, 2015, http://www.npr.org/sections/health-shots/2015/08/04 /428164731/is-obamacares-research-institute-worth-the-billions.

76. Nicholas Bagley, "Who Says PCORI Can't Do Cost Effectiveness?" *The Incidental Economists: A Health Services Research Blog*, October 14, 2013, http://theincidentaleconomist.com/wordpress/who-says-pcori-cant-do-cost-effectiveness/.

77. Fred Schulte, "Is Obamacare's Research Institute Worth the Billions?"

78. Ibid.

79. Eric Patashnik, "Here Are the 5 Reasons Republicans Are Trying to Cut Research on Evidence-Based Medicine," *Washington Post*, October 22, 2015, https://www.washingtonpost.com/news/monkey-cage/wp/2015/06/22/here-are -the–5-reasons-republicans-are-trying-to-cut-research-on-evidence-based -medicine/?utm_term=.c0543444b649; Schulte, "Is Obamacare's Research Institute Worth the Billions?"

80. Casey Ross, "This Federal Agency That Aims to Make Health Care More Effective Is on the Chopping Block, Again," STAT, March 30, 2017, https://www .statnews.com/2017/03/30/ahrq-budget-trump-nih/.

81. James D. Chambers, M. J. Cangelosi, and P. J. Neumann, "Medicare's Use of Cost-Effectiveness Analysis for Prevention (But Not for Treatment)," *Health Policy* 119, no. 2 (2015): 156–63; P. A. Deverka and J. C. Dreyfus, "Clinical Integration of Next-Generation Sequencing: Coverage and Reimbursement Challenges," *Journal of Law, Medicine & Ethics* 42, Suppl. 1 (2014): 22–41; A. M. Garber, "Evidence-Based Coverage Policy," *Health Affairs* 20, no. 5 (2001): 62–82; A. Hresko and S. B. Haga, "Insurance Coverage Policies for Personalized Medicine," *Journal of Personalized Medicine* 2 (2012): 201–16; J. R. Trosman, S. L. Van Bebber, and K. A. Phillips, "Health Technology Assessment and Private Payers' Coverage of Personalized Medicine," *Journal of Oncology Practice* 7 (3S) (2011): 18s–24s.

82. R. A. Rettig, et al., *False Hope: Bone Marrow Transplantation for Breast Cancer* (New York: Oxford University Press, 2007); Sorenson, et al., "The Politics of Comparative Effectiveness Research: Lessons from Recent History."

83. Health Care Financing Administration, "Medicare Program; Criteria and Procedures for Making Medical Services Coverage Decisions That Relate to Health Care Technology," *Federal Register* 54, no. 18 (1989): 4302, at 4308.

84. Ibid.

85. S. B. Foote, "Why Medicare Cannot Promulgate a National Coverage Rule: A Case of Regula Mortis," *Journal of Health Politics, Policy, and Law* 27 (2002): 707–30; Neumann et al., "Medicare and Cost-Effectiveness Analysis."

86. Neumann, et al., "Medicare and Cost-Effectiveness Analysis."

87. Robin J. Strongin, "Medicare Coverage: Lessons from the Past, Questions for the Future," National Issues Forum Background Paper, August 2001, http:// www.nhpf.org/library/background-papers/BP_MedicareCoverage_8–01.pdf.

88. Foote, "Why Medicare Cannot Promulgate a National Coverage Rule: A Case of Regula Mortis."

89. Sean R. Tunis and Steven D. Pearson, "Coverage Options for Promising Technologies: Medicare's Coverage with Evidence Development," *Health Affairs* 25, no. 5 (2006): 1218–30.

90. Bryan Luce and Rebecca Singer Cohen, "Health Technology Assessment in the United States."

91. Rita F. Redberg and Judith Walsh, "Pay Now, Benefits May Follow—The Case of Cardiac Computed Tomographic Angiography," *New England Journal of Medicine* 359 (2008): 2309–11.

92. P. J. Neumann and J. Chambers, "Medicare's Reset on 'Coverage with Evidence Development,'" *Health Affairs Blog*, April 1, 2013, http://healthaffairs.org/blog/2013/04/01/medicares-reset-on-coverage-with-evidence-development/.

93. Ibid.

94. James C. Robinson, "Applying Value-Based Insurance Design to High-Cost Health Services," *Health Affairs* 29, no. 11 (2010): 2009–16.

95. Margaret O'Kane, "Increasing Transparency on Health Care Costs, Coverage, and Quality," Testimony before the Senate Commerce, Science & Transportation Committee, February 27, 2013.

96. Brian Elbel and Mark Schlesinger, "Responsive Consumerism: Empowerment in Markets for Health Plans," *The Milbank Quarterly* 87, no. 3 (2009): 633–82.

97. Bruce C. Vladeck, et al., "Consumers and Hospital Use: The HCFA 'Death List,'" *Health Affairs* 7, no. 1 (1988): 122–25.

98. Andrew J. Epstein, "Do Cardiac Surgery Report Cards Reduce Mortality? Assessing the Evidence," *Medical Care Research and Review* 63, no. 4 (2006): 403–26; D. H. Howard, "Quality and Consumer Choice in Healthcare: Evidence from Kidney Transplantation," *Topics in Economic Analysis and Policy* 5, no. 1 (2005): 1–20.

99. Garber, "Evidence-Based Coverage Policy."

100. Linda A. Bergthold, "Medical Necessity: Do We Need It?" *Health Affairs* 14, no. 4 (1995): 180–90.

101. Ibid.

102. V. Lo Re, et al., "Disparities in Absolute Denial of Modern Hepatitis C Therapy by Type of Insurance," *Clinical Gastroenterology and Hepatology* 14, no. 7 (2016): 1035–43.

Chapter 3

1. Paul Starr, *Remedy and Reaction: The Peculiar American Struggle over Health Care Reform, Revised Edition* (New Haven, CT: Yale University Press, 2013).

2. Breastcancer.org, www.breastcancer.org.

3. National Cancer Institute, Surveillance, Epidemiology, and End Results Program, https://seer.cancer.gov/.

4. American Cancer Society, https://www.cancer.org.

5. Breastcancer.org, www.breastcancer.org.

6. Ismail Jatoi and Anthony B. Miller, "Why Is Breast Cancer Mortality Declining?" *The Lancet Oncology* 4, no. 4 (2003): 251–54.

7. Michael K. Gusmano, Victor G. Rodwin, and Daniel Weisz, "Persistent Inequalities in Health and Access to Health Services: Evidence from NYC," *World Medical & Health Policy*, 9, no. 2 (2017): 186–205.

8. Gopal K. Singh and Ahmedin Jemal, "Socioeconomic and Racial/Ethnic Disparities in Cancer Mortality, Incidence, and Survival in the United States, 1950–2014: Over Six Decades of Changing Patterns and Widening Inequalities," *Journal of Environmental and Public Health*, 2017; https://doi.org/10.1155/2017 /2819372, https://www.hindawi.com/journals/jeph/2017/2819372/abs/.

9. Bijou R. Hunt, Steve Whitman, and Marc S. Hurlbert, "Increasing Black: White Disparities in Breast Cancer Mortality in the 50 Largest Cities in the United States," *Cancer Epidemiology* 38, no. 2 (2014): 118–23.

10. Singh and Jemel, "Socioeconomic and Racial/Ethnic Disparities in Cancer Mortality, Incidence, and Survival in the United States, 1950–2014: Over Six Decades of Changing Patterns and Widening Inequalities."

11. American Cancer Society, 2016, https://www.cancer.org/latest-news/nih -to-fund-study-of-breast-cancer-in-black-women.html.

12. Julia B. Corbett and Motomi Mori, "Medicine, Media, and Celebrities: News Coverage of Breast Cancer, 1960–1995," *Journalism and Mass Communication Quarterly* 76, no. 2 (1999): 229–49.

13. *Our Bodies, Ourselves*, https://www.ourbodiesourselves.org/publications /our-bodies-ourselves-2011/introduction/.

14. Corbett and Mori, "Medicine, Media, and Celebrities: News Coverage of Breast Cancer, 1960–1995."

15. Janice Hopkins Tanne, "Celebrity Illnesses Raise Awareness, But Can Give Wrong Message," *BMJ* 321, no. 7369 (2000): 1099.

16. Baron Lerner, *Breast Cancer Wars: Hope, Fear, and the Pursuit of a Cure in Twenty-First Century America* (Oxford: Oxford University Press, 2001).

17. Vicki Brower, "The Squeaky Wheel Gets the Grease," *EMBO Reports* 6, no. 11 (2005): 1014–17.

18. Susan Braun, "The History of Breast Cancer Advocacy," *The Breast Journal* 9(s2) (2003): S101–S103; Bob Riter, "A Very Brief History of the Breast Cancer Advocacy Movement," 2008, http://www.cancerlynx.com/breastadvocacy.html.

19. Brower, "The Squeaky Wheel Gets the Grease," 1016.

20. Maureen Hogan Casamayou, *The Politics of Breast Cancer* (Washington, D.C.: Georgetown University Press, 2001); Maureen Hogan Casamayou, "Review of the Breast Cancer Wars: Hope, Fear, and the Pursuit of a Cure in Twentieth-Century America," *Journal of Health Politics, Policy and Law* 27, no. 6 (2002): 1037–39; Patricia Strach, *Hiding Politics in Plain Sight: Cause Marketing, Corporate Influence, and Breast Cancer Policymaking* (New York: Oxford University Press, 2016).

21. Ibid.

22. Ibid.

23. A. C. Keller and L. Packel, "Going for the Cure: Patient Interest Groups and Health Advocacy in the United States," *Journal of Health Politics, Policy, and Law* 39, no. 2 (2014): 331–67.

24. Lea Goldman, "The Big Business of Breast Cancer," *MarieClaire*, September 14, 2011, http://www.marieclaire.com/politics/news/a6506/breast-cancer-business-scams/.

25. J. R. Ashley and Cecine N. Nguyen, "A Comparison of Cancer Burden and Research Spending Reveals Discrepancies in the Distribution of Research Funding," *BMC Public Health* 12 (2012): 526.

26. Nicholas Wilcken, "How Breast Cancer Treatment Has Evolved Since the 1950s," *American Council on Society and Health*, June 1, 2016, https://www.acsh.org/news/2016/06/01/how-breast-cancer-treatment-has-evolved-since-the-1950s.

27. Stefan Aebi, et al., "Chemotherapy for Isolated Locoregional Recurrence of Breast Cancer: The CALOR Randomised Trial," *Lancet Oncology* 15, no. 2 (2014): 156–63; George W. Sledge, et al., "Past, Present, and Future Challenges in Breast Cancer Treatment," *Journal of Clinical Oncology* 32, no. 19 (2014): 1979–86.

28. Charlotte Grayson, "New Approaches to Chemotherapy for Breast Cancer," MedicineNet.com, September 7, 2002, http://www.medicinenet.com/script/main/art.asp?articlekey=51886.

29. Aura Muntasell, et al., "Interplay between Natural Killer Cells and Anti-HER2 Antibodies: Perspectives for Breast Cancer Immunotherapy," *Frontiers in Immunology* 8 (2017): 1544. doi: 10.3389/fimmu.2017.01544DOI=10.3389/fimmu.2017.01544.

30. Richard H. Gold, Lawrence W. Bassett, and Bobbi Widoff, "Highlights from the History of Mammography," *Radiographics* 10 (1990): 1111–31.

31. Gold, et al., "Highlights from the History of Mammography."

32. Robert L. Egan. "Fifty-Three Cases of Carcinoma of the Breast: Occult Until Mammography," *American Journal of Roentgenology* 88 (1962): 1095–1101.

33. Jane Wells, "Mammography Screening and the Politics of Randomised Trials," *BMJ* 317, no. 7172 (1998): 1224–30.

34. Lydia E. Pace and Nancy L. Keating, "A Systematic Assessment of Benefits and Risks to Guide Breast Cancer Screening Decisions," *Journal of the American Medical Association* 311, no. 13 (2014): 1327–35.

35. Pace and Keating, "A Systematic Assessment of Benefits and Risks to Guide Breast Cancer Screening Decisions."

36. E. R. Myers, et al., "Benefits and Harms of Breast Cancer Screening: A Systematic Review," *Journal of the American Medical Association* 314, no. 15 (2015): 1615–34.

37. Gold, "Highlights from the History of Mammography."

38. Cornelia J. Baines, "Rational and Irrational Issues in Breast Cancer Screening," *Cancers* 3, no. 1 (2011): 252–66.

39. Baines, "Rational and Irrational Issues in Breast Cancer Screening"; E. Lidbrink, J. Elfving, and E. Jonsonn, "Neglected Aspects of False Positive Findings of Mammography in Breast Cancer Screening: Analysis of False Positive Cases from the Stockholm Trial," *BMJ* 312 (1996): 273–76.

40. Gail R. Wilensky, "The Mammography Guidelines and Evidence-Based Medicine," *Health Affairs Blog*, January 12, 2010, https://www.healthaffairs.org /do/10.1377/hblog20100112.003427/full/.

41. Virginia L. Ernster, "Mammography Screening for Women Aged 40 through 49—A Guidelines Saga," *American Journal of Public Health* 87, no. 7 (1997): 1103–06.

42. Lidbrink, et al., "Neglected Aspects of False Positive Findings of Mammography in Breast Cancer Screening: Analysis of False Positive Cases from the Stockholm Trial."

43. Ernster, "Mammography Screening for Women Aged 40 through 49—A Guidelines Saga and a Clarion Call for Informed Decision Making."

44. S. Woloshin, et al., "Cancer Screening Campaigns—Getting Past Uninformative Persuasion," *New England Journal of Medicine* 367, no. 18 (2012): 1677–79.

45. Mette Kalager, et al., "Failure to Account for Selection Bias," *International Journal of Cancer* 113, no. 11 (2013): 2751–53.

46. Alexandra Sifferlin, "Breast Cancer Screening: How Komen Oversold the Benefits of Mammography," *Time*, August 3, 2012, http://healthland.time.com /2012/08/03/breast-cancer-screening-komen-ad-overstated-the-benefits-of -mammography-researchers-say/.

47. J. Hirschman, S. Whitman, and D. Ansell, "The Black: White Disparity in Breast Cancer Mortality: The Example of Chicago," *Cancer Causes & Control* 18, no. 3 (2007): 323–33.

48. W. D. den Brok, et al., "Survival with Metastatic Breast Cancer Based on Initial Presentation, De Novo versus Relapsed," *Breast Cancer Research and Treatment* 161, no. 3 (2017): 549–56.

49. Anne H. Partridge and Eric P. Winer, "On Mammography—More Agreement Than Disagreement," *New England Journal of Medicine* 361, no. 26 (2009): 2499–2501.

50. Jatoi and Miller, "Why Is Breast Cancer Mortality Declining?"

51. Archie Bleyer and H. Gilbert Welch, "Effect of Three Decades of Screening Mammography on Breast Cancer Incidence," *New England Journal of Medicine* 367, no. 21 (2012): 1998–2005.

52. Peggy Eastman, "NCI Adopts New Mammography Screening Guidelines for Women," *Journal of the National Cancer Institute* 89, no. 8 (1997): 538–50.

53. Ernster, "Mammography Screening for Women Aged 40 through 49—A Guidelines Saga and a Clarion Call for Informed Decision Making."

54. National Institutes of Health Consensus Development Panel, "National Institutes of Health Consensus Development Conference Statement: Breast Cancer Screening for Women Ages 40–49, January 21–23, 1997," *JNCI: Journal of the National Cancer Institute* 89, no. 14 (1997): 960–65.

55. National Institutes of Health Consensus Development Panel, "National Institutes of Health Consensus Development Conference Statement: Breast Cancer Screening for Women Ages 40–49, January 21–23, 1997."

56. U.S. Senate, Mammography: Hearings before a Subcommittee of the Committee on Appropriations, United States Senate, One Hundred Fifth Congress, First Session. Special Hearings (Washington, D.C.: Government Printing Office, 1997), https://www.gpo.gov/fdsys/pkg/CHRG–105shrg44044/html/CHRG–105shrg44044.htm.

57. Ibid.

58. Ibid.

59. Eastman, "NCI Adopts New Mammography Screening Guidelines for Women."

60. Lerner, *Breast Cancer Wars: Hope, Fear, and the Pursuit of a Cure in Twenty-First Century America.*

61. Section 2713 of the Patient Protection and Affordable Care Act, 42 U.S.C. § 18001, 2010.

62. N. Calonge, et al., "Screening for Breast Cancer: U.S. Preventive Services Task Force Recommendation Statement," *Annals of Internal Medicine* 151, no. 10 (2009): 716–26.

63. Ibid.

64. Ibid., 717.

65. Ibid., 718.

66. HemOne Today, "USPSTF Breast Cancer Screening Recommendations Remain Unchanged Despite Controversy," *HemOne Today*, January 11, 2016, https://www.healio.com/hematology-oncology/breast-cancer/news/in-the-journals/%7B4e79de36-911d-41ef-bed3-3ad171be2f26%7D/uspstf-breast-cancer-screening-recommendations-remain-unchanged-despite-controversy.

67. Ibid.

68. Jeanne Lenzer, "Is the United States Preventive Services Task Force Still a Voice of Caution?" *BMJ* 356 (2017): j743 doi: 10.1136/bmj.j743.

69. Uwe E. Reinhardt, "The Uproar Over Mammography," Economix, Explaining the Science of Everyday Life. *The New York Times*, November 20, 2009.

70. Wilensky, "The Mammography Guidelines and Evidence-Based Medicine."

71. Reinhardt, "The Uproar Over Mammography."

72. Wilensky, "The Mammography Guidelines and Evidence-Based Medicine."

73. The Wall Street Journal, "Liberals and Mammography: Rationing? What Rationing? Review and Outlook," *The Wall Street Journal Online*, November 24, 2009, https://www.wsj.com/articles/SB10001424052748704779704574552320222125990.

74. Ernster, "Mammography Screening for Women Aged 40 through 49—A Guidelines Saga and a Clarion Call for Informed Decision Making."

75. Susan G. Komen for the Cure® Scientific Advisory Board's Perspective on the U.S. Preventive Services Task Force (USPSTF) Recommendations on Breast Screening, November 2009, https://ww5.komen.org/ResearchAndGrants/Perspective-OnUSPSTFRecommendationsOnScreening.aspx.

76. Transcript: Dr. Bernadine Healy on *FNS*, November 23, 2009, http://www.foxnews.com/story/2009/11/23/transcript-dr-bernadine-healy-on-fns.html.

77. UPI, "Sebelius: Mammogram Policies Unchanged," UPI Top News, November 18, 2009, https://www.upi.com/Top_News/US/2009/11/18/Sebelius -Mammogram-policies-unchanged/UPI-18271258591793/.

78. David M. Herszenhorn, "Senate Blocks the Use of New Mammography Guidelines," *New York Times*, December 3, 2009, https://prescriptions.blogs .nytimes.com/2009/12/03/gop-amendments-aim-at-new-cancer-guidelines/.

79. Bradford H. Gray, Michael K. Gusmano, and Sara Collins, "AHCPR and the Politics of Health Services Research," *Health Affairs—Web Exclusive*, 2003, W3283– W307, https://s3.amazonaws.com/academia.edu.documents/39679961/AHCPR _and_the_Changing_Politics_of_Healt20151104-22646-1hdvtk4.pdf?AWSAccess KeyId=AKIAIWOWYYGZ2Y53UL3A&Expires=1515977474&Signature=T4qIJzc9j 3wt2JlY4A09adyVFpo%3D&response-content-disposition=inline%3B%20 filename%3DAHCPR_And_The_Changing_Politics_Of_Healt.pdf.

80. Committee on Ways and Means, Subcommittee on Health, U.S. House of Representatives, *MEDPAC Report on Medicare Payment Policies*. Hearing, One Hundred Eighth Congress, First Session, March 6. Serial. no. 108–14 (Washington, D.C.: U.S. Government Printing Office, 2003).

81. Adam G. Elshaug, et al., "Challenges in Australian Policy Processes for Disinvestment from Existing, Ineffective Health Care Practices," *Australia and New Zealand Health Policy* 4 (2007): 23.

82. Daniel Béland, "Reconsidering Policy Feedback: How Policies Affect Politics," *Administration & Policy* 42, no. 5 (2010): 568–90.

83. Uwe Reinhardt, "Divide et Impera: Protecting the Growth Health Care Incomes (COSTS)," *Health Economics* 21, no. 1 (2012): 41–54.

84. Daniel Kahneman and Amos Tversky, "Advances in Prospect Theory: Cumulative Representation of Uncertainty," *Journal of Risk and Uncertainty* 5, no. 4 (1992): 297–323.

85. Daniel Callahan, *Taming the Beloved Beast: How Medical Technology Is Ruining Our Health System* (Oxford: Oxford University Press, 2009).

86. Strach, *Hiding Politics in Plain Sight: Cause Marketing, Corporate Influence, and Breast Cancer Policymaking*.

87. Virginia Hopkins, "Mammogram Controversy—Follow the Money," *Health Watchers' News and Views*, November 18, 2009, http://www.healthwatch-ersnews.com/2009/11/mammogram-controversy-follow-the-money/.

88. Alicia Mundy, "New Breast Screening Limits Face Reversal," *The Wall Street Journal*, January 12, 2010, https://www.wsj.com/articles/SB1263257 63413725559.

89. Ibid.

90. Wilensky, "The Mammography Guidelines and Evidence-Based Medicine."

91. Nortin Hadler, "Does Screening Mammography Save Lives?" *ABC News*, May 21, 2007, http://abcnews.go.com/Health/OnCallPlus/story?id=3196417.

92. Samantha King, *Pink Ribbons, Inc.: Breast Cancer and the Politics of Philanthropy* (Minneapolis: University of Minnesota Press, 2006); Strach, *Hiding Politics in Plain Sight: Cause Marketing, Corporate Influence, and Breast Cancer Policymaking*.

93. Strach, *Hiding Politics in Plain Sight: Cause Marketing, Corporate Influence, and Breast Cancer Policymaking*.

94. Ibid.

95. King, *Pink Ribbons, Inc.: Breast Cancer and the Politics of Philanthropy*; Strach, *Hiding Politics in Plain Sight: Cause Marketing, Corporate Influence, and Breast Cancer Policymaking*.

96. Michael K. Gusmano, Mark Schlesinger, and Tracey Thomas, "Policy Feedback and Public Opinion: The Role of Employer Responsibility in Social Policy," *Journal of Health Politics, Policy, and Law* 27, no. 5 (2002): 731–72.

97. King, *Pink Ribbons, Inc.: Breast Cancer and the Politics of Philanthropy*; Strach, *Hiding Politics in Plain Sight: Cause Marketing, Corporate Influence, and Breast Cancer Policymaking*.

98. Strach, *Hiding Politics in Plain Sight: Cause Marketing, Corporate Influence, and Breast Cancer Policymaking*.

99. King, *Pink Ribbons, Inc.: Breast Cancer and the Politics of Philanthropy*.

100. National Cancer Institute, http://www.cancer.gov/cancertopics/high-dose -chemo.

101. Kerianne H. Quanstrum and Rodney A. Hayward, "Lessons from the Mammography Wars," *New England Journal of Medicine* 363, no. 11 (2010): 1076–79.

102. Adam Finkel, "Disinfecting Evidence-Based Policy Analysis of Hidden Value-Laden Constraints," *The Hastings Center Report* 48, no. 1 (2018): S21–S49.

103. Thomas Coburn, "Majority's Health Bill Empowers Government Task Force at Center of Mammogram Controversy," 2009, from website of Senator Tom Coburn (R-OK), http://coburn.library.okstate.edu/right_now/2009/12/senate-health-care -bill-costs-taxpayers-6-8-million-per-word.html.

104. American Cancer Society, https://www.cancer.org/content/dam/cancer-org/ research/cancer-facts-and-statistics/breast-cancer-facts-and-figures/breast-cancer -facts-and-figures-2017-2018.pdf.

105. Coburn, "Majority's Health Bill Empowers Government Task Force at Center of Mammogram Controversy."

106. *Wall Street Journal*, "Liberals and Mammography. Rationing? What Rationing?"

107. Patient Protection and Affordable Care Act, 42 U.S.C. § 18001, 2010.

108. Ibid.

109. Health Care and Education Reconciliation Act of 2010 (H.R. 4872).

110. Daniel Callahan, "Controlling Costs: Do as Business Does," *Health Care Cost Monitor*, January 29, 2009; Elliott S. Fisher, Julie P. Bynum, and Jonathan S. Skinner, "Slowing the Growth of Health Care Costs—Lessons from Regional Variation," *New England Journal of Medicine* 360, no. 9 (2009): 849–52; Theodore Marmor, Jonathan Oberlander, and Joseph White, "The Obama Administration's Options for Health Care Cost Control: Hope Versus Reality," *Annals of Internal Medicine* 150, no. 7 (2009): 485–89.

111. Michael F. Cannon, "A Better Way to Generate and Use Comparative-Effectiveness Research," *Policy Analysis* 632 (2009): 1–21; M. Chassin, "Variations in the Use of Medical and Surgical Services by the Medicare Population," *New England Journal of Medicine* 314, no. 5 (1986): 285–90; Fisher, et al., "Slowing the Growth of Health Care Costs—Lessons from Regional Variation"; John K.

Iglehart, "Prioritizing Comparative-Effectiveness Research—IOM Recommendations," *New England Journal of Medicine* 361, no. 4 (2009): 325–28.

112. Fisher, et al., "Slowing the Growth of Health Care Costs—Lessons from Regional Variation."

113. Patient Protection and Affordable Care Act, 42 U.S.C. § 18001, 2010.

Chapter 4

1. CMS, https://www.medicare.gov/what-medicare-covers/index.html.

2. Jonathan Oberlander, *The Political Life of Medicare* (Chicago: University of Chicago Press, 2003), 123.

3. Ibid., 119–11.

4. S. R. Kaufman and L. Fjord, "Medicare, Ethics, and Reflexive Longevity," *Medical Anthropology Quarterly* 25, no. 2 (2011): 209–31, at 217.

5. Daniel Callahan, *Taming the Beloved Beast: How Medical Technology Is Ruining Our Health System* (Oxford: Oxford University Press, 2009).

6. Oberlander, *The Political Life of Medicare*, 123.

7. Social Security Act Sec. 1862, 42 U.S.C. 1395y (a) (1)(A).

8. Alzheimer's Association, https://www.alz.org/alzheimers_disease_what _is_alzheimers.asp.

9. CMS, "Decision Memo for Beta Amyloid Positron Emission Tomography in Dementia and Neurodegenerative Disease (CAG-0431N)," September 27, 2013, https://www.cms.gov/medicare-coverage-database/details/nca-decision-memo .aspx?NCAId=265.

10. Ibid.

11. Alzheimer's Association, "What Is Dementia?" https://www.alz.org/what -is-dementia.asp.

12. Ibid.

13. Marilyn S. Albert, et al. "The Diagnosis of Mild Cognitive Impairment Due to Alzheimer's Disease: Recommendations from the National Institute on Aging-Alzheimer's Association Workgroups on Diagnostic Guidelines for Alzheimer's Disease," *Alzheimer's & Dementia* 7, no. 3 (2011): 270–79; Clifford R. Jack, et al., "Introduction to the Recommendations from the National Institute on Aging-Alzheimer's Association Workgroups on Diagnostic Guidelines for Alzheimer's Disease," *Alzheimer's & Dementia* 7, no. 3 (2011): 257–62; Guy M. McKhann, et al., "The Diagnosis of Dementia Due to Alzheimer's Disease: Recommendations from the National Institute on Aging-Alzheimer's Association Workgroups on Diagnostic Guidelines for Alzheimer's Disease," *Alzheimer's & Dementia* 7, no. 3 (2011): 263–69;

14. Jason Karlawish, "Addressing the Ethical, Policy, and Social Challenges of Preclinical Alzheimer Disease," *Neurology* 77, no. 15 (2011): 1487–93.

15. Alzheimer's Association, "Alzheimer's Disease Facts and Figures," 2015, https://www.alz.org/facts/downloads/facts_figures_2015.pdf.

16. CMS, "Decision Memo for Beta Amyloid Positron Emission Tomography in Dementia and Neurodegenerative Disease (CAG-0431N)."

17. Ibid.

18. Lilly USA, LLC, Request for Reconsideration of Medical National Coverage Determinations Manual, § 220.6, Positron Emission Tomography (PET) Scans, 2012, https://www.cms.gov/Medicare/Coverage/DeterminationProcess /downloads/id265.pdf.

19. Food & Drug Administration, Approval Package for Florbetapir F 18 Injection, April 6, 2012, https://www.accessdata.fda.gov/drugsatfda_docs/nda /2012/202008Orig1s000Approv.pdf.

20. CMS, "Decision Memo for Beta Amyloid Positron Emission Tomography in Dementia and Neurodegenerative Disease (CAG-0431N)."

21. MITA, "About MITA," https://www.medicalimaging.org/about-mita/.

22. Susan Bartlett Foote, "Why Medicare Cannot Promulgate a National Coverage Rule: A Case of Regula Mortis," *Journal of Health Politics, Policy, and Law* 27, no. 5 (2002): 707–30; Susan Bartlett Foote, "Focus on Locus: Evolution of Medicare's Local Coverage Policy," *Health Affairs* 22, no. 4 (2003): 137–46; M. R. Gillick, "Medicare Coverage for Technological Innovations—Time for New Criteria?" *New England Journal of Medicine* 350 (2004): 2199–2203.

23. James D. Chambers, et al. "Changing Face of Medicare's National Coverage Determinations for Technology," *International Journal of Technology Assessment in Health Care* 31, no. 5 (2016): 1–8.

24. Susan Bartlett Foote, et al., "Resolving the Tug-of-War between Medicare's National and Local Coverage," *Health Affairs* 23, no. 4 (2004): 108–23; Office of Inspector General, U.S. Department of Health and Human Services, "Local Coverage Determinations Create Inconsistency in Medicare Coverage," January 7, 2014, http://oig.hhs.gov/oei/reports/oei-01-11-00500.pdf.

25. Chambers, et al., "Changing Face of Medicare's National Coverage Determinations for Technology"; Peter J. Neumann and Sean R. Tunis, "Medicare and Medical Technology—The Growing Demand for Relevant Outcomes," *New England Journal of Medicine* 362, no. 5 (2010): 377–79.

26. Office of Inspector General, "Local Coverage Determinations Create Inconsistency in Medicare Coverage."

27. Foote, "Why Medicare Cannot Promulgate a National Coverage Rule: A Case of Regula Mortis."

28. Health Care Financing Administration, Medicare Program, "Criteria for Making Coverage Decisions," *Federal Register* 65, no. 95 (2000): 31124–29, at 31127.

29. CMS, "Medicare Program; Revised Process for Making National Determinations," *Federal Register* 78, no. 152 (August 7, 2013): 48164–69.

30. Hansel Javier Otero, et al., "Medicare's National Coverage Determinations in Diagnostic Radiology: Examining Evidence and Setting Limits," *Academic Radiology* 19, no. 9 (2012): 1060–65.

31. J. D. Chambers, K. E. May, and P. J. Neumann, "Medicare Covers the Majority of FDA-Approved Devices and Part B Drugs, but Restrictions and Discrepancies Remain," *Health Affairs* 32, no. 6 (2013): 1109–15; J. D. Chambers, et al., "Medicare Is Scrutinizing Evidence More Tightly for National Coverage

Determinations," *Health Affairs* 34, no. 2 (2015): 253–60; Chambers, et al., "Changing Face of Medicare's National Coverage Determinations for Technology."

32. Chambers, et al., "Medicare Covers the Majority of FDA-Approved Devices and Part B Drugs, but Restrictions and Discrepancies Remain."

33. Foote, "Why Medicare Cannot Promulgate a National Coverage Rule: A Case of Regula Mortis"; Sandra J. Carnahan, "Medicare's Coverage with Study Participation Policy: Clinical Trials or Tribulations," *Yale Journal of Health Policy Law & Ethics* 7, no. 2 (2007): 229–72.

34. Gina Kolata, "Medicare Covering New Treatments with a Catch," *New York Times*, November 5, 2004, http://query.nytimes.com/gst/fullpage.html?res=9A02E3DF153CF936A35752C1A9629C8B63&pagewanted=all.

35. CMS, "Decision Memo for Beta Amyloid Positron Emission Tomography in Dementia and Neurodegenerative Disease (CAG-0431N)," 15.

36. Stéphane Lavertu, Daniel E. Walters, and David L. Weimer, "Scientific Expertise and the Balance of Political Interests: MEDCAC and Medicare Coverage Decisions," *Journal of Public Administration Research and Theory* 22, no. 1 (2011): 55–81, at 61.

37. Ibid.

38. CMS, Medicare Evidence Development & Coverage Advisory Committee, "Beta Amyloid Positron Emission Tomography (PET) in Dementia and Neurodegenerative Disease," January 30, 2013, https://www.cms.gov/medicare-coverage-database/details/medcac-meeting-details.aspx?MEDCACId=66.

39. Keith A. Johnson, et al., "Appropriate Use Criteria for Amyloid PET: A Report of the Amyloid Imaging Task Force, the Society of Nuclear Medicine and Molecular Imaging, and the Alzheimer's Association," *Journal of Nuclear Medicine* 54, no. 3 (2013): 476–90; Keith A. Johnson, et al., "Update on Appropriate Use Criteria for Amyloid PET Imaging: Dementia Experts, Mild Cognitive Impairment, and Education," *Journal of Nuclear Medicine* 54, no. 7 (2013): 1011–13.

40. Bruce J. Hillman, Richard A. Frank, and Brian C. Abraham, "The Medical Imaging & Technology Alliance Conference on Research Endpoints Appropriate for Medicare Coverage of New PET Radiopharmaceuticals," *Journal of Nuclear Medicine* 54, no. 9 (2013): 1675–79.

41. Bruce J. Hillman, Richard A. Frank, and Gail M. Rodriguez, "New Pathways to Medicare Coverage for Innovative PET Radiopharmaceuticals: Report of a Medical Imaging & Technology Alliance (MITA) Workshop," *Journal of Nuclear Medicine* 53, no. 2 (2012): 336–42.

42. Ibid., 338.

43. Foote, "Focus on Locus: Evolution of Medicare's Local Coverage Policy."

44. Ibid., 338; Liz Richardson, "Aligning FDA and CMS Review," *Health Affairs Policy Brief*, August 27, 2015, 10.1377/hpb20150827.132391, https://www.healthaffairs.org/do/10.1377/hpb20150827.132391/full/.

45. Hillman, et al. "New Pathways to Medicare Coverage for Innovative PET Radiopharmaceuticals: Report of a Medical Imaging & Technology Alliance (MITA) Workshop."

46. Ibid., 338.

47. Ibid., 338.

48. Hillman, et al. "The Medical Imaging & Technology Alliance Conference on Research Endpoints Appropriate for Medicare Coverage of New PET Radio-pharmaceuticals," 1675.

49. Ibid., 1678.

50. ALZ Forum, "Coverage Denial for Amyloid Scans Riles Alzheimer's Community," July 25, 2013, http://www.alzforum.org/news/conference-coverage /coverage-denial-amyloid-scans-riles-alzheimers-community.

51. S. Molchan, "A Tale of Two Conferences," *Journal of the American Medical Association Internal Medicine* 174, no. 6 (2014): 856–57.

52. Ibid.

53. Public Citizen, "RE: Proposed Decision Memo for Beta Amyloid Positron Emission Tomography in Dementia and Neurodegenerative Disease (CAG-0043IN)," July 23, 2013.

54. Robert Steinbrook, "The Centers for Medicare & Medicaid Services and Amyloid-β Positron Emission Tomography for Alzheimer Disease," *Journal of the American Medical Association Internal Medicine* 174, no. 1 (2014): 135.

55. B. W. Mol, et al., "Characteristics of Good Diagnostic Tests," *Seminars in Reproductive Medicine* 21, no. 1 (2003): 17–25.

56. D. G. Fryback and J. R. Thornbury, "The Efficacy of Diagnostic Imaging," *Medical Decision Making* 11, no. 2 (1991): 88–94.

57. CMS, "Decision Memo for Beta Amyloid Positron Emission Tomography in Dementia and Neurodegenerative Disease (CAG-0431N)," 18.

58. Ibid.

59. Ibid.

60. Ibid.

61. Ibid., 1.

62. Lilly, "Lilly Disappointed in Medicare Decision to Deny Appropriate Patient Access to Beta-Amyloid Imaging Agents, Including Amyvid™ (Florbetapir F 18 Injection), Despite Support from Experts, Patients, and the Alzheimer's Disease Community," September 27, 2013, https://investor.lilly.com/releasedetail .cfm?releaseid=793700.

63. E. Silverman, "Lilly Backs Lawsuit Against CMS Over Its Alzheimer's Diagnostic Drug," *Wall Street Journal*, September 5, 2014, http://blogs.wsj.com/pharma-lot/2014/09/05/lilly-backs-lawsuit-against-cms-over-its-alzheimers-diagnostic-drug/.

64. *Smith v. Burwell*, No. 14-1519. U. S. District Court for the District of Columbia, September 4, 2014.

65. Silverman, "Lilly Backs Lawsuit Against CMS Over Its Alzheimer's Diagnostic Drug."

66. *Kort v. Burwell*, U.S. District Court for the District of Columbia, 209 F. Supp.3d 98 (2016), p. 118.

67. Ibid.

68. ALZFORUM, "Alzheimer's Community Mobilizes to Show Benefits of Amyloid Scans," October 11, 2013, https://www.alzforum.org/news/community -news/alzheimers-community-mobilizes-show-benefits-amyloid-scans.

69. IDEAS. "Imaging Dementia—Evidence for Amyloid Scanning," https://www.ideas-study.org/about/history/.

70. Hillman, et al. "New Pathways to Medicare Coverage for Innovative PET Radiopharmaceuticals: Report of a Medical Imaging & Technology Alliance (MITA) Workshop."

71. IDEAS, "Protocol," https://www.ideas-study.org/referring-physicians /protocol/, 19.

72. Ibid., p. 9.

73. IDEAS, https://www.ideas-study.org/.

74. IDEAS, "Interim Results from the IDEAS Study Reported at AAIC 2017 in London," https://www.ideas-study.org/2017/07/20/interim-results-from-the -ideas-study-reported-at-aaic-2017-in-london/.

75. Ibid.

76. David Blumenthal, Karen Davis, and Stuart Guterman, "Medicare at 50— Origins and Evolution," *New England Journal of Medicine* 372, no. 7 (2015): 671–77; Jonathan Oberlander, *The Political Life of Medicare*.

77. Peter J. Neumann and Sean R. Tunis, "Medicare and Medical Technology—The Growing Demand for Relevant Outcomes," *New England Journal of Medicine* 362, no. 5 (2010): 377–79.

78. Ibid., 377.

79. Chambers, et al., "Medicare is Scrutinizing Evidence More Tightly for National Coverage Determinations."

80. Chambers, et al., "Medicare Covers the Majority of FDA-Approved Devices and Part B Drugs, but Restrictions and Discrepancies Remain."

81. Hansel Javier Otero, James D. Chambers, Brian W. Bresnahan, Maki S. Kamae, Kent E. Yucel, and Peter J. Neumann," Medicare's National Coverage Determinations in Diagnostic Radiology: Examining Evidence and Setting Limits," *Academic Radiology* 19, no. 9 (2012): 1060–65.

82. J. D. Chambers, P. J. Neumann, and M. J. Buxton, "Does Medicare Have an Implicit Cost-Effectiveness Threshold?" *Medical Decision Making* 30 (2010): E14–E27.

83. C. Sorenson, M. K. Gusmano, and A. Oliver, "The Politics of Comparative Effectiveness Research: Lessons from Recent History," *Journal of Health Politics, Policy, and Law* 39, no. 1 (2014): 139–70.

84. D. B. Kramer and A. S. Kesselheim, "Coverage of Magnetic Resonance Imaging for Patients with Cardiac Devices: Improving the Coverage with Evidence Development Program," *Journal of the American Medical Association Cardiology* 2 (2017): 711–12.

85. Foote, "Why Medicare Cannot Promulgate a National Coverage Rule: A Case of Regula Mortis."

86. Gillick, "Coverage for Technological Innovations—Time for New Criteria?"

Chapter 5

1. Food & Drug Administration, "FDA Approves Sovaldi for Chronic Hepatitis C," *FDA News Release*, December 9, 2013, https://www.hhs.gov/hepatitis/blog/2013/12/09/fda-approves-sovaldi-for-chronic-hepatitis-c.html.

2. Centers for Disease Control and Prevention, "Hepatitis C FAQs for the Public," https://www.cdc.gov/hepatitis/hcv/cfaq.htm#cFAQ35

3. A. G. Singal, et al., "A Sustained Viral Response Is Associated with Reduced Liver Related Morbidity and Mortality in Patients with Hepatitis C Virus," *Clinical Gastroenterology and Hepatology* 8 (2010): 280–88, 288.e1; S. Sarkar, et al., "Fatigue Before, During, and After Antiviral Therapy of Chronic Hepatitis C: Results from the Virahep-C Study," *Journal of Hepatology* 57 (2012): 946–52; L. I. Backus, et al., "A Sustained Virologic Response Reduces Risk of All-Cause Mortality in Patients with Hepatitis C," *Clinical Gastroenterology and Hepatology* 9 (2011): 509–16, e1.; A. J. van der Meer, et al., "Association Between Sustained Virological Response and All-Cause Mortality Among Patients with Chronic Hepatitis C and Advanced Hepatic Fibrosis," *Journal of the American Medical Association* 308 (2010): 2584–93; K. Rutter, et al., "Successful Antiviral Treatment Improves Survival of Patients with Advanced Liver Disease Due to Chronic Hepatitis C," *Alimentary Pharmacology & Therapeutics* 41 (2015): 521–31.

4. Stacey B. Trooskin, Helen Reynolds, and Jay R. Kostman, "Access to Costly New Hepatitis C Drugs: Medicine, Money, and Advocacy," *Clinical Infectious Diseases* 61, no. 2 (2015): 1825–30.

5. Centers for Disease Control and Prevention, "Hepatitis C FAQs for the Public."

6. Ibid.

7. L. Schiff, "Finding Truth in a World Full of Spin: Myth-Busting in the Case of Sovaldi," *Clinical Therapeutics* 37, no. 5 (2015): 1092–1112.

8. E. W. Chak, S. Sarkar, and C. Bowlus, "Improving Healthcare Systems to Reduce Healthcare Disparities in Viral Hepatitis," *Digestive Diseases and Sciences* 61, no. 10 (2016); 2776–83.

9. Ibid.

10. Beth Snyder Bulik, "Gilead Pushes Hep C Testing in Baby Boomers as Its Blockbusters Plummet," *FiercePharma*, February 22, 2017, https://www.fiercepharma.com/marketing/baby-boomers-targeted-gilead-hepatitis-c-awareness-campaign-even-as-drug-s-fortunes-drop.

11. Chak, Sarkar, and Bowlus, "Improving Healthcare Systems to Reduce Healthcare Disparities in Viral Hepatitis."

12. Michael Ollove, "Are States Obligated to Provide Expensive Hepatitis C Drugs?" *The PEW Charitable Trusts*, February 9, 2016, http://www.pewtrusts.org/en/research-and-analysis/blogs/stateline/2016/02/09/are-states-obligated-to-provide-expensive-hepatitis-c-drugs.

13. Chak, Sarkar, and Bowlus, "Improving Healthcare Systems to Reduce Healthcare Disparities in Viral Hepatitis."

14. Ibid.

15. Ibid., 2780.

16. Trooskin, Reynolds, and Kostman, "Access to Costly New Hepatitis C Drugs: Medicine, Money, and Advocacy," 1825.

17. Anne Schneider and Helen Ingram, "Social Construction of Target Populations: Implications for Politics and Policy," *American Political Science Review* 87, no. 2 (1993): 334–47.

18. Nicholas J. Burstow, et al., "Hepatitis C Treatment: Where Are We Now?" *International Journal of General Medicine* 10 (2017): 39–52.

19. M. P. Manns, H. Wedemeyer, and M. Cornber, "Treating Viral Hepatitis C: Efficacy, Side Effects, And Complications," *Gut* 55 (2006): 1350–59.

20. Bernard Sanders, "Opening Statement. Hepatitis C and Veterans," Hearing before the Committee on Veterans' Affairs, One Hundred Thirteenth Congress, Second Session, December 3, 2014.

21. Manns, Wedemeyer, and Cornber, "Treating Viral Hepatitis C: Efficacy, Side Effects, and Complications."

22. Sanders, "Opening Statement. Hepatitis C and Veterans."

23. Burstow, "Hepatitis C Treatment: Where Are We Now?"

24. Reuters Staff, "FDA Approves Gilead's Breakthrough Hepatitis C Pill," Reuters, December 6, 2013, https://www.reuters.com/article/us-gilead-fda-hepatitis/fda-approves-gileads-breakthrough-hepatitis-c-pill-idUSBRE9B 50YB20131206.

25. Food & Drug Administration, Drug Approval Package, Harvoni, https://www.accessdata.fda.gov/drugsatfda_docs/nda/2014/205834Orig1s000TOC .cfm; Gilead, "U.S. Food and Drug Administration Approves Gilead's Harvoni® (Ledipasvir/Sofosbuvir), the First Once-Daily Single Tablet Regimen for the Treatment of Genotype 1 Chronic Hepatitis C," https://www.gilead.com/news /press-releases/2014/10/us-food-and-drug-administration-approves-gileads -harvoni-ledipasvirsofosbuvir-the-first-oncedaily-single-tablet-regimen-for -the-treatment-of-genotype-1-chronic-hepatitis-c.

26. Ibid.

27. Carolyn Y. Johnson and Brady Dennis, "How an $84,000 Drug Got Its Price: 'Let's Hold Our Position . . . Whatever the Headlines,'" *Washington Post*, December 1, 2015, https://www.washingtonpost.com/news/wonk/wp/2015 /12/01/how-an-84000-drug-got-its-price-lets-hold-our-position-whatever-the -headlines/?utm_term=.cc34a100501d.

28. Ollove, "Are States Obligated to Provide Expensive Hepatitis C Drugs?"

29. Schiff, "Finding Truth in a World Full of Spin: Myth-Busting in the Case of Sovaldi."

30. Virgil Dickson, "Reform Update: Medicaid Programs Crafting Limits on Harvoni Usage," *Modern Healthcare*, October 21, 2014, http://www.modernhealthcare.com /article/20141021/NEWS/310219962.

31. Ollove, "Are States Obligated to Provide Expensive Hepatitis C Drugs?"

32. Dickson, "Reform Update: Medicaid Programs Crafting Limits on Harvoni Usage."

33. Sony Salzman, "How Insurance Providers Deny Hepatitis C Patients Life-saving Drugs," *Al Jazeera America*, October 19, 2015, http://america.aljazeera .com/articles/2015/10/16/insurance-providers-deny-hepatitis-drugs.html.

34. Amber M. Charles, "Indifference, Interruption, and Immunodeficiency: The Impact and Implications of Inadequate HIV/AIDS Care in U.S. Prisons," *Boston University Law Review* 92, no. 6 (2012): 1979–2022.

35. Ibid.

36. Adam Beckman, et al., "New Hepatitis C Drugs Are Very Costly and Unavailable to Many State Prisoners," *Health Affairs* 35, no. 10 (2017): 1893–1901.

37. *Hoffer et al. v. Jones*, U.S. District Court for the Northern District of Florida. Case 4:17-cv-00214-MW-CAS Document 185, Filed December 13, 2017.

38. Michelle Andrews, "FDA's Approval of a Cheaper Drug for Hepatitis C Will Likely Expand Treatment," NPR, October 4, 2017, https://www.npr.org /sections/health-shots/2017/10/04/555156577/fdas-approval-of-a-cheaper-drug -for-hepatitis-c-will-likely-expand-treatment.

39. Peter S. Arno and Michael H. Davis, "The New Face of US Health Care: $1,000 per Pill," *Truthout*, December 23, 2014, http://www.truth-out.org/opinion/item /28171-the-new-face-of-us-health-care-1-000-per-pill.

40. Chatwal Jagpreet, et al., "Cost-Effectiveness and Budget Impact of Hepatitis C Virus Treatment with Sofosbuvir and Ledipasvir in the United States," *Annals of Internal Medicine* 162, no. 6 (2015): 397–406. doi:10.7326/M14-1336.

41. Arno and Davis, "The New Face of US Health Care: $1,000 per Pill."

42. Ollove, "Are States Obligated to Provide Expensive Hepatitis C Drugs?"

43. Ibid.

44. Trooskin, "Access to Costly New Hepatitis C Drugs: Medicine, Money, and Advocacy."

45. Centers for Disease Control and Prevention, "Hepatitis C FAQs for the Public."

46. Michael K. Gusmano and Mark Schlesinger, "The Social Roles of Medicare: Assessing Medicare's Collateral Benefits," *Journal of Health, Politics, Policy, and Law* 26, no. 1 (2001): 37–81.

47. UNAIDS. "90-90-90: An Ambitious Treatment Target to Help End the AIDS Epidemic," Joint United Nations Programme on HIV/AIDS (UNAIDS), October 2014.

48. Patient-Centered Outcomes Research Institute. "Can CER Help Answer Questions about Hepatitis C? A PCORI Stakeholder Workshop," May 18, 2016, https://www.pcori.org/events/2016/can-cer-help-answer-questions-about -hepatitis-c-pcori-stakeholder-workshop.

49. Margaret Weir, Ann Shola Orloff, and Theda Skocpol, *The Politics of Social Policy in the United States* (Princeton, NJ: Princeton University Press, 1988).

50. Ollove, "Are States Obligated to Provide Expensive Hepatitis C Drugs?"

51. Liz Szabo, "Breakthrough Cancer Drug Could Be Astronomical in Price," *USA Today*, August 22, 2017, https://www.usatoday.com/story/news/2017/08/22 /breakthrough-cancer-drug-astronomical-price/589442001/.

52. Salzman, "How Insurance Providers Deny Hepatitis C Patients Lifesaving Drugs."

53. Andrews, "FDA's Approval of a Cheaper Drug for Hepatitis C Will Likely Expand Treatment."

54. Ollove, "Are States Obligated to Provide Expensive Hepatitis C Drugs?"

55. Andrews, "FDA's Approval of a Cheaper Drug for Hepatitis C Will Likely Expand Treatment."

56. Hep Magazine, "Missouri Is the Latest State to Roll Back Restrictions on Hepatitis C Treatment," Hep Magazine, December 1, 2017, https://www.hepmag.com/article/missouri-latest-state-roll-back-restrictions-hepatitis-c-treatment.

57. Ibid.

58. Schiff, "Finding Truth in a World Full of Spin: Myth-Busting in the Case of Sovaldi."

59. Andrews, "FDA's Approval of a Cheaper Drug for Hepatitis C Will Likely Expand Treatment."

60. Laurie Toich, "Will Hepatitis C Virus Medication Costs Drop in the Years Ahead?" *Pharmacy Times*, February 8, 2017, http://www.pharmacytimes.com/resource-centers/hepatitisc/will-hepatitis-c-virus-medicaton-costs-drop-in-the-years-ahead.

61. Tracy Staton, "Gilead and Express Scripts Make Peace in Hep C with 2017 Formulary Deal," FiercePharma, December 15, 2016. https://www.fiercepharma.com/pharma/gilead-and-express-scripts-make-peace-hep-c-2017-formulary-deal.

62. Paul Kleutghen, et al., "Drugs Don't Work if People Can't Afford Them: The High Price of Tisagenlecleucel," *Health Affairs Blog*, February 8, 2018, https://www.healthaffairs.org/do/10.1377/hblog20180205.292531/full/; Karen J. Maschke, Michael K. Gusmano, and Mildred Z. Solomon, "Expensive Breakthrough Treatments: The Case of CAR-T Cell Cancer Treatment," *Health Affairs* 36, no. 10 (2017): 1698–1700.

63. Maschke, Gusmano, and Solomon, "Expensive Breakthrough Treatments: The Case of CAR-T Cell Cancer Treatment."

64. Donald J. Trump, "President Donald J. Trump's State of the Union Address," The White House, January 30, 2018, https://www.whitehouse.gov/briefings-statements/president-donald-j-trumps-state-union-address/.

65. Panos Kanavos, et al., "Higher US Branded Drug Prices and Spending Compared to Other Countries May Stem Partly from Quick Uptake of New Drugs," *Health Affairs* 32, no. 4 (2013): 753–61.

66. OECD, "OECD Health Statistics 2014: How Does the United States Compare?", http://www.oecd.org/unitedstates/Briefing-Note-UNITED-STATES–2014.pdf.

67. Marcia Angell, *The Truth About Drug Companies: How They Deceive Us and What to Do About It* (New York: Random House, 2005).

68. Ollove, "Are States Obligated to Provide Expensive Hepatitis C Drugs?"

69. John LaMattina, "Gilead's CEO Admits to 'Failures' in Setting Price of $1,000-a-Pill Breakthrough," Forbes, December 8, 2016, https://www.forbes.com/sites/johnlamattina/2016/12/08/gileads-ceo-apologetic-about-sovaldis-1000-per-pill-price-tag/#6d58bc431a97.

70. Arno and Davis, "The New Face of US Health Care: $1,000 per Pill."

71. Gerard F. Anderson, B. K. Frogner, and Uwe Reinhardt, "Health Spending in OECD Countries in 2004: An Update," *Health Affairs* 26, no. 5 (2007): 1481–89; Joseph White, "Prices, Volume, and the Perverse Effects of the Variations Crusade," *Journal of Health Politics, Policy, and Law* 36, no. 4 (2011): 775–90.

72. Salzman, "How Insurance Providers Deny Hepatitis C Patients Lifesaving Drugs."

73. Jagpreet, et al., "Cost-Effectiveness and Budget Impact of Hepatitis C Virus Treatment with Sofosbuvir and Ledipasvir in the United States."

74. David Meltzer and James Magnus, "Inconsistencies in the 'Societal Perspective' on Costs of the Panel on Cost-Effectiveness in Health and Medicine," *Medical Decision Making* 19, no. 4 (1999): 371–77.

75. Leonard B. Saltz, "Can Money Really Be No Object When Cancer Care Is the Subject?" *Journal of Clinical Oncology* 33, no. 10 (2015): 1093–94.

76. Thomas C. Schelling, "The Life You Save May Be Your Own," in *Problems in Public Expenditure Analysis,* ed. S. B. Chaase (Washington, D.C.: The Brookings Institution, 1968), 127–176.

77. Michael K. Gusmano, et al., "Health Care as an Investment? Reframing the Health Policy Debates in Europe," *Alliance for Health & the Future,* Issue Brief 3, no. 1 (2008): 1–7; http://researchonline.lshtm.ac.uk/7463/1/Health%20Care%20 as%20an%20Investment%20Reframing%20the%20Health%20Policy%20 Debates%20in%20Europe.pdf.

78. S. H. Woolf, et al., *The Economic Argument for Disease Prevention: Distinguishing Between Value and Savings.* A Prevention Policy Paper Commissioned by Partnership for Prevention, 2009: 5.

79. New England Healthcare Institute, *Balancing Act: Comparative Effectiveness Research and Innovation in U.S. Health Care,* A White Paper, April 2009: 2.

80. Arno and Davis, "The New Face of US Health Care: $1,000 per Pill."

81. Ibid.

82. Uwe Reinhardt, "Probing Our Moral Values in Health Care: The Pricing of Specialty Drugs," *Journal of the American Medical Association* 314, no. 10 (2015): 981–82.

83. Arno and Davis, "The New Face of US Health Care: $1,000 per Pill."

Chapter 6

1. Aaron S. Kesselheim, "Trends in Utilization of FDA Expedited Drug Development and Approval Programs, 1987–2014: Cohort Study," *BMJ* 351 (2015): h4633. doi: https://doi.org/10.1136/bmj.h4633.

2. General Accountability Office, "DRUG SAFETY: FDA Expedites Many Applications, but Data for Postapproval Oversight Need Improvement," Report to the Ranking Member, Subcommittee on Labor, Health and Human Services, Education, and Related Agencies, Committee on Appropriations, House of Representatives, GAO–16–1 (Washington, D.C.: General Accountability Office, 2015).

3. Richard Harris, "R&D Costs for Cancer Drugs Are Likely Much Less than Industry Claims, Study Finds," NPR, WNYC Radio, September 11, 2017, https:// www.npr.org/sections/health-shots/2017/09/11/550135932/r-d-costs-for-cancer -drugs-are-likely-much-less-than-industry-claims-study-finds.

4. Public Citizen, "Rx R&D Myths: The Case Against the Drug Industry's R&D 'Scare Card,'" Congress Watch, July 2001, https://www.citizen.org/sites /default/files/rdmyths.pdf.

5. Aaron S. Kesselheim, et al., "Existing FDA Pathways Have Potential to Ensure Early Access to, and Appropriate Use of Specialty Drugs," *Health Affairs* 30, no. 10 (2014): 1770–78.

6. Rob Stein, "FDA Considers Revoking Approval of Avastin for Advanced Breast Cancer," *Washington Post*, August 16, 2010, http://www.washingtonpost. com/wp-dyn/content/article/2010/08/15/AR2010081503466.html.

7. James G. Dickinson, "It's Time to Replace the FDA, Says Newt Gingrich," MM&N, May 1, 2014, https://www.mmm-online.com/legalregulatory/its-time -to-replace-the-fda-says-newt-gingrich/article/343560/.

8. Sheila Kaplan, "Trump Derides 'Slow and Burdensome' Approval Process at FDA," STAT, February 28, 2017, https://www.statnews.com/2017/02/28/trump -address-rare-disease-drugs/.

9. Adam Feuerstein, "Trump's FDA May Be Lowering the Standards for Drug Approvals. What's the Fallout?" STAT, July 11, 2017, https://www.statnews .com/2017/07/11/trump-fda-gottlieb-standards/.

10. Adam Feuerstein, "Shift in Drug Approval Process at FDA Under Trump? Here & Now," WBUR 90.9, July 12, 2017, http://www.wbur.org/hereandnow/2017 /07/12/drug-approval-process-fda-trump.

11. T. Shih and C. Lindley, "Bevacizumab: An Angiogenesis Inhibitor for the Treatment of Solid Malignancies," *Clinical Therapeutics* 28, no. 11 (2006): 1779–1802.

12. K. J. Gotink and H. M. Verheul, "Anti-Angiogenic Tyrosine Kinase Inhibitors: What Is Their Mechanism of Action?" *Angiogenesis* 13, no. 1 (2010): 1–14.

13. H. X. Chen and J. N. Cleck, "Adverse Effects of Anticancer Agents that Target the VEGF Pathway," *Nature Reviews Clinical Oncology* 6, no. 8 (2009): 464–77.

14. Samuel Hopkins Adams, "The Great American Fraud: Articles on the Nostrum Evil and Quacks, in Two Series," Reprinted by *Collier's Weekly*, 4th edition (New York: P.F. Collier & Son, 1911).

15. Marc Law and Gary D. Libecap, "The Determinants of Progressive Era Reform. The Pure Food and Drugs Act of 1906," in *Corruption and Reform: Lessons from America's Economic History*, eds. Edward L. Glaeser and Claudia Goldin (Chicago: University of Chicago Press, 2006), 319–41.

16. Pure Food and Drug Act of 1906, Public Law 59-384.

17. David F. Cavers, "The Food, Drug, and Cosmetic Act of 1938: Its Legislative History and Its Substantive Provisions," *Law and Contemporary Problems* 6, no. 1 (1939): 2–42.

18. Ibid.

19. Ibid., 9.

20. Food & Drug Administration History, September 29, 2017, https://www .fda.gov/AboutFDA/WhatWeDo/History/.

21. Federal Food, Drug, and Cosmetic Act (June 25, 1938, ch. 675, § 1, 52 Stat. 1040).

22. Food & Drug Administration History.

23. Act of October 10, 1962 (Drug Amendments Act of 1962), Public Law 87-781, 76 Stat. 780.

24. David A. Kessler, "The Regulation of Investigational Drugs," *New England Journal of Medicine* 320, no. 5 (1989): 281–88, at 283.

25. Bruce J. Hillman, *A Plague on All Our Houses: Medical Intrigue, Hollywood, and the Discovery of AIDS* (Lebanon, NH: ForeEdge, 2016).

26. Steven Epstein, *Impure Science: AIDS, Activism, and the Politics of Knowledge* (Berkeley: University of California Press, 1996), 3.

27. Ibid.

28. Rebecca Dresser, *When Science Offers Salvation: Patient Advocacy and Research Ethics* (New York: Oxford University Press, 2001).

29. Kesselheim, et al., "Existing FDA Pathways Have Potential to Ensure Early Access to, and Appropriate Use of, Specialty Drugs."

30. Michael Henry Davis, Peter S. Arno, and Karen Bonuck, "Rare Diseases, Drug Development, and AIDS: The Impact of the Orphan Drug Act," Law Faculty Articles and Essays, Cleveland State University, 1995.

31. Kesselheim, "Trends in Utilization of FDA Expedited Drug Development and Approval Programs, 1987–2014: Cohort Study."

32. Ibid., 351.

33. Michael McCaughan, "Health Policy Brief: Expedited Approval Pathways," *Health Affairs*, July 21, 2017, doi: 10.1377/hpb2017.2

34. Kesselheim, et al., "Existing FDA Pathways Have Potential to Ensure Early Access to, and Appropriate Use of, Specialty Drugs."

35. Food & Drug Administration, "Hearing on Proposal to Withdraw Approval for the Breast Cancer Indication for Bevacizumab (Avastin)" (Washington, D.C.: U.S. Department of Health and Human Services), July 6, 2011, https://www.fda.gov/NewsEvents/MeetingsConferencesWorkshops/ucm 255874.htm.

36. McCaughan, "Health Policy Brief: Expedited Approval Pathways."

37. Food and Drug Administration Safety and Innovation Act of 2012, Public Law 112-144.

38. Kesselheim, "Trends in Utilization of FDA Expedited Drug Development and Approval Programs, 1987–2014: Cohort Study."

39. General Accountability Office, "DRUG SAFETY: FDA Expedites Many Applications, but Data for Postapproval Oversight Need Improvement."

40. Ibid.

41. M. H. Cohen, et al., "FDA Drug Approval Summary: Bevacizumab (Avastin) Plus Carboplatin and Paclitaxel as First-Line Treatment of Advanced/Metastatic Recurrent Nonsquamous Non-Small-Cell Lung Cancer," *Oncologist* 12, no. 6 (2007): 713–18.

42. M. Reck, et al., "Overall Survival with Cisplatin-Gemcitabine and Bevacizumab or Placebo as First-Line Therapy for Nonsquamous Non-Small-Cell Lung Cancer: Results from a Randomised Phase III trial (AVAiL)," *Annals of Oncology* 21, no. 9 (2010): 1804–09.

43. A. Vitry, et al., "Regulatory Withdrawal of Medicines Marketed with Uncertain Benefits: The Bevacizumab Case Study," *Journal of Pharmaceutical Policy and Practice* 8 (2015): 25.

44. Ibid.

45. Richard Pazdur, "Memorandum to the File BLA 125085 Avastin (bevacizumab): Regulatory Decision to Withdraw Avastin (bevacizumab) First-Line Metastatic Breast Cancer Indication." FDA Center For Drug Evaluation And Research, 2010, https://www.fda.gov/downloads/Drugs/DrugSafety/PostmarketDrug SafetyInformationforPatientsandProviders/UCM237171.pdf.

46. Ibid.

47. Vitry, et al., "Regulatory Withdrawal of Medicines Marketed with Uncertain Benefits: The Bevacizumab Case Study."

48. Lee Pai-Scherf and Lu Hong, "STN 125085/91 Bevacizumab (Avastin®) plus Paclitaxel for First-Line Metastatic Breast Cancer: Clinical Review," ODAC Meeting, December 5, 2007, https://www.fda.gov/ohrms/dockets/ac/07/slides /2007–4332s1–02-FDA-Pai-Scherf-Lu.ppt.

49. Ibid.

50. Pazdur, "Memorandum to the File BLA 125085 Avastin (bevacizumab): Regulatory Decision to Withdraw Avastin (bevacizumab) First-Line Metastatic Breast Cancer Indication."

51. Food & Drug Administration [Docket No. FDA–2010–N–0621], "Proposal to Withdraw Approval for the Breast Cancer Indication for Bevacizumab; Hearing," May 11, 2011, *Federal Register* 86, no. 91, 27332–35, https://www.gpo.gov /fdsys/pkg/FR–2011–05–11/pdf/2011–11539.pdf#page=1.

52. Pazdur, "Memorandum to the File BLA 125085 Avastin (bevacizumab): Regulatory Decision to Withdraw Avastin (bevacizumab) First-Line Metastatic Breast Cancer Indication."

53. Vitry, et al., "Regulatory Withdrawal of Medicines Marketed with Uncertain Benefits: The Bevacizumab Case Study."

54. Food & Drug Administration, "Hearing on Proposal to Withdraw Approval for the Breast Cancer Indication for Bevacizumab (Avastin)."

55. Ibid.

56. Ibid.

57. Valarie Blake, "The Terminally Ill, Access to Investigational Drugs, and FDA Rules," *AMA Journal of Ethics* 15, no. 8 (2013): 687–91.

58. Food & Drug Administration, "Hearing on Proposal to Withdraw Approval for the Breast Cancer Indication for Bevacizumab (Avastin)."

59. M. Herper, "The FDA's Cancer Czar Says He Can't Approve New Drugs Fast Enough," *Forbes*, June 23, 2013, www.forbes.com/sites/matthewherper/2013/06/23 /the-fdas-cancer-czarsays-he-cant-approve-new-drugs-fast-enough/.

60. Donald W. Light and Joel Lexchin, "Why Do Cancer Drugs Get Such an Easy Ride? *BMJ* 2015;350:h2068, doi:10.1136/bmj.h2068.

61. Food & Drug Administration, "Hearing on Proposal to Withdraw Approval for the Breast Cancer Indication for Bevacizumab (Avastin)," 50.

62. Ibid., 46.

63. Christopher M. Booth, and Elizabeth A. Eisenhauer, "Progression-Free Survival: Meaningful or Simply Measurable?" *Journal of Clinical Oncology* 30, no. 10 (2012): 1030–33.

64. Food & Drug Administration, "Hearing on Proposal to Withdraw Approval for the Breast Cancer Indication for Bevacizumab (Avastin)."

65. S. Michiels, E. D. Saad, and M. Buyse, "Progression-Free Survival as a Surrogate for Overall Survival in Clinical Trials of Targeted Therapy in Advanced Solid Tumors," *Drugs* 77, no. 7 (2017): 713–19.

66. Thomas R. Fleming, "Surrogate Endpoints and FDA's Accelerated Approval Process: The Challenges Are Greater than They Seem," *Health Affairs* 24, no. 1 (2005): 67–78.

67. Ibid.

68. Booth and Eisenhauer, "Progression-Free Survival: Meaningful or Simply Measurable?", 1030.

69. Vinay Prasad, "Perspective: The Precision-Oncology Illusion," *Nature* 537, no. 7619 (2016): S63; Tito Fojo, "Precision Oncology: A Strategy We Were Not Ready to Deploy," *Seminars in Oncology* 43, no. 1 (2016): 9–12.

70. Vinay Prasad and A. Vandross, "Characteristics of Exceptional or Super Responders to Cancer Drugs," *Mayo Clinic Proceedings* 90, no. 12 (2015): 1639–49.

71. Andrew Pollack, "Breast Cancer Patients Plead for Avastin Approval," *New York Times*, June 28, 2011, http://www.nytimes.com/2011/06/29/business/29drug.html.

72. Food & Drug Administration, "Hearing on Proposal to Withdraw Approval for the Breast Cancer Indication for Bevacizumab (Avastin)," 56.

73. Ibid., 88.

74. Ibid., 20–21.

75. Ibid., 75.

76. Ibid., 33.

77. Ibid., 43.

78. Ibid., 83.

79. Thomas M. Burton and Jennifer Corbett Dooren, "Key FDA Approval Yanked for Avastin," *Wall Street Journal*, November 19, 2011, https://www.wsj.com/articles/SB10001424052970203699404577046041941288780.

80. Daniel Carpenter, "Strengthen and Stabilize the FDA," *Nature* 485: 169–70.

Chapter 7

1. Pedro M. Baptista and Anthony Atala, "Regenerative Medicine: The Hurdles and Hopes," in *Translating Regenerative Medicine to the Clinic*, eds., Jeffrey Laurence, Pedro M. Baptista and Anthony Atala (Amsterdam: Elsevier, 2016), 1–7, at 3.

2. Jane Maienschein, "Regenerative Medicine's Historical Roots in Regeneration, Transplantation, and Translation," *Developmental Biology* 358, no. 2 (2011): 278–84.

3. Alliance for Regenerative Medicine, "Industry Overview," https://alliancerm.org/page/industry-overview.

4. National Institutes of Health, "Stem Cell Basics, https://stemcells.nih.gov/info/basics.htm.

5. National Research Council and Institute of Medicine, *Stem Cells and the Future of Regenerative Medicine* (Washington, D.C.: National Academies Press, 2002), 8.

6. Darren Lau, et al., "Stem Cell Clinics Online: The Direct-to-Consumer Portrayal of Stem Cell Medicine," *Cell Stem Cell* 3, no. 6 (2008): 591–94.

7. 21 U.S.C. 9, §321 (g)(1).

8. 42 U.S.C. §247d.

9. Food & Drug Administration, Human Cells Tissues, and Cellular and Tissue-Based Products, *Federal Register* 55, no. 5447 (January 19, 2001), 5448.

10. Food & Drug Administration, Human Cells Tissues, and Cellular and Tissue-Based Products, *Federal Register* 55, no. 5447 (January 19, 2001), 5458; (codified at 21 CFR 1271).

11. Ibid., 5467.

12. Ibid.

13. Ibid., 5457.

14. *U.S. vs. Regenerative Sciences*, 848 F. Supp. 2d 248 (2012).

15. Patients for Stem Cells, http://patientsforstemcells.org/; Christen Rachul, "'What Have I Got to Lose?' An Analysis of Stem Cell Therapy Patients' Blogs," *Health Law Review* 20, no. 1 (2011): 5–12; Emily Ramshaw, "Perry's Surgery Included Experimental Stem Cell Therapy," *Texas Tribune*, August 3, 2011, https://www.texastribune.org/2011/08/03/perrys-surgery-included-experimental-stem-cell-the/.

16. Karen J. Maschke and Michael K. Gusmano, "Evidence and Access to Biomedical Interventions: The Case of Stem Cell Treatments," *Journal of Health Politics, Policy, and Law* 41, no. 5 (2016): 917–36; Ramshaw, "Perry's Surgery Included Experimental Stem Cell Therapy."

17. Katherine Drabiak-Syed, "Challenging the FDA's Authority to Regulate Autologous Adult Stem Cells for Therapeutic Use: Celltex Therapeutics' Partnership with RNL Bio, Substantial Medical Risks, and the Implications of *United States v. Regenerative Sciences*," *Health Matrix* 23 (2013): 493–535, at 498.

18. David Cyranoski, "Stem-cell Therapy Takes off in Texas," *Nature*, 483, no. 738 (2012): 13-15; Drabiak-Syed, "Challenging the FDA's Authority to Regulate Autologous Adult Stem Cells for Therapeutic Use: Celltex Therapeutics' Partnership with RNL Bio, Substantial Medical Risks, and the Implications of *United States v. Regenerative Sciences*," 498.

19. Susan Berfield, "Stem Cell Showdown: Celltex versus the FDA," Bloomberg Businessweek, January 3, 2013, http://www.businessweek.com/articles/2013–01–03/stem-cell-showdown-celltex-vs-dot-the-fda.

20. Ramshaw, "Perry's Surgery Included Experimental Stem Cell Therapy."

21. Katherine Drabiak-Syed, "Challenging the FDA's Authority to Regulate Autologous Adult Stem Cells for Therapeutic Use: Celltex Therapeutics' Partnership with RNL Bio, Substantial Medical Risks, and the Implications of *United States v. Regenerative Sciences*."

22. Ibid.

23. David B. Cyranoski, "Stem Cells in Texas: Cowboy Culture," *Nature* 494, no. 7436 (2013): 166–68.

24. Celltex, http://celltexbank.com/.

25. *U.S. vs. Regenerative Sciences*, Civ. Action No. 10-1327 (RMC), Memorandum Opinion, July 23, 2012.

26. Jeffrey K. Shapiro, "FDA to Hold a Public Hearing for a Quartet of Draft HCT/P Guidances: A Scorecard," November 2, 2015, FDA Law Blog, http://www .fdalawblog.net/2015/11/fda-to-hold-a-public-hearing-for-a-quartet-of-draft-hctp -guidances-a-scorecard/.

27. Food & Drug Administration, "Same Surgical Procedure Exception under 21 CFR 1271.15(b): Questions and Answers Regarding the Scope of the Exception," Draft Guidance, October 2014, 4.

28. Food & Drug Administration, "Human Cells, Tissues, and Cellular and Tissue-Based Products (HCT/Ps) from Adipose Tissue: Regulatory Considerations," Draft Guidance for Industry, December 2014, 3.

29. Food & Drug Administration, "Minimal Manipulation of Human Cells, Tissues, and Cellular and Tissue-Based Products," Draft Guidance for Industry and Food and Drug Administration Staff, December 2014, 8.

30. Food & Drug Administration, Final Agenda, Part 15 Hearing, September 12–13, 2016, https://www.fda.gov/biologicsbloodvaccines/newsevents/workshop smeetingsconferences/ucm509279.htm; Transcript, Part 15 Hearing, "Draft Guidances Relating to the Regulation of Human Cells, Tissues or Cellular Products," September 12, 2016, https://www.fda.gov/downloads/Biologics BloodVaccines/NewsEvents/WorkshopsMeetingsConferences/UCM532350 .pdf; September 13, 2016, https://www.fda.gov/downloads/BiologicsBlood Vaccines/NewsEvents/WorkshopsMeetingsConferences/UCM532633 .pdf.

31. Leigh Turner and Paul Knoepfler, "Selling Stem Cells in the USA: Assessing the Direct-to-Consumer Industry," *Cell Stem Cell* 19, no. 2 (2016): 154–57.

32. Food & Drug Administration, "Public Workshop. Scientific Evidence in Development of HCT/Ps Subject to Premarket Approval," September 8, 2016, https://www.fda.gov/downloads/BiologicsBloodVaccines/NewsEvents/Workshops MeetingsConferences/UCM530238.pdf; Irving Weissman, "Stem Cell Therapies Could Change Medicine . . . If They Get the Chance," *Cell Stem Cell* 10, no. 6 (2012): 663–65.

33. Laura Beil, "Stem Cell Treatments Overtake Science," *New York Times*, September 9, 2013, http://www.nytimes.com/2013/09/10/health/stem-cell-treatments-overtake-science.html; Leigh Turner, "US Stem Cell Clinics, Patient Safety, and the FDA," *Trends in Molecular Medicine* 21, no. 5 (2015): 271–73; Weissman, "Stem Cell Therapies Could Change Medicine . . . If They Get the Chance."

34. Amy Scharf and Elizabeth Dzeng, "'I'm Willing to Try Anything': Compassionate Use Access to Experimental Drugs and the Misguided Mission of Right-to-Try Laws," *Health Affairs Blog*, March 27, 2017, https://www.healthaffairs.org/do/10.1377/hblog20170327.059378/full/.

35. Christina Corieri, "Everyone Deserves the Right to Try: Empowering the Terminally Ill to Take Control of Their Treatment," Goldwater Institute, February 11, 2014, https://goldwaterinstitute.org/wp-content/uploads/cms_page_media/2015/1/29/Right%20To%20Try.pdf.

36. Morgan Griffith, "Congressman Griffith's Weekly E-Newsletter 5.5.14," https://morgangriffith.house.gov/news/documentsingle.aspx?DocumentID=378942.

37. Elizabeth Richardson, et al., "Right-to-Try Laws," Health Policy Brief, *Health Affairs*, April 9, 2015, http://www.healthaffairs.org/healthpolicybriefs/brief.php?brief_id=135; Kelly Servick, "'Right to Try' Laws Bypass FDA for Last-Ditch Treatments, *Science* 344, no. 6190 (2014): 1329.

38. Paul Knoepfler, "Neuralstem Flirting with Stem Cell Noncompliance in Colorado via Right to Try Law?" *The Niche, Knoepfler Lab Stem Cell Blog*, June 11, 2014, https://ipscell.com/2014/06/neuralstem-flirting-with-stem-cell-noncompliance-in-colorado-via-right-to-try-law/.

39. Kelly Servick, "Texas Has Sanctioned Unapproved Stem Cell Therapies. Will It Change Anything?" *Science*, June 15, 2017, http://www.sciencemag.org/news/2017/06/texas-has-sanctioned-unapproved-stem-cell-therapies-will-it-change-anything; H.B. 810. http://www.capitol.state.tx.us/tlodocs/85R/billtext/pdf/HB00810E.pdf#navpanes=0.

40. Courtney Friedman, "Gov. Abbott Signs HB 810, Allowing Texans to Use Own Stem Cells as Medicine, www.KSAT.com, June 13, 2017, https://www.ksat.com/news/politics/gov-abbott-signs-hb–810-allowing-texans-to-use-own-stem-cells-as-medicine.

41. Kelly Servick, "Texas Has Sanctioned Unapproved Stem Cell Therapies. Will it Change Anything?"

42. Trickett Wendler, et al., "Right to Try Act of 2017," https://www.congress.gov/bill/115th-congress/senate-bill/204.

43. Sarah Karlin-Smith and Seung Min Kim, "Senate Approves 'Right-to-Try' Drug Bill," August 3, 2017, Politico, https://www.politico.com/story/2017/08/03/senate-right-to-try-drug-bill-241293.

44. Scott Gottlieb, "Examining Patient Access to Investigational Drugs," Testimony before the Subcommittee on Health, Committee on Energy and Commerce, U.S. House of Representatives, October 3, 2017, https://www.fda.gov/NewsEvents/Testimony/ucm578634.htm.

45. Ibid.

46. Erin Mershon, "Pence Says that Congress Should Get Right-to-Try Legislation 'DONE,'" STAT, January 18, 2018, https://www.statnews.com/2018/01/18/mike-pence-right-to-try/.

47. Ibid.

48. Ike Swetlitz, "In State of Union, Trump Endorses 'Right to Try' For Terminally Ill Patients," STAT, January 30, 2018, https://www.statnews.com/2018/01/30/state-of-the-union-trump-right-to-try/.

49. "Donnelly and Chairman of House Energy and Commerce Committee Discuss Bipartisan Efforts to Accelerate Medical Breakthroughs," Joe Donnelly,

United States Senator for Indiana, November 16, 2015, https://www.donnelly
.senate.gov/newsroom/press/donnelly-and-chairman-of-house-energy-and
-commerce-committee-discuss-bipartisan-efforts-to-accelerate-medical
-breakthroughs.

50. Sam Stein, Ryan Grim, and Matt Fuller, "Congress Is About to Pass a Bill
that Shows D.C. at Its Worst—It May Also Turn Around the Opioid Crisis and
Cure Cancer," Huffington Post, November 29, 2016, https://www.huffingtonpost
.com/entry/congress-21st-century-cures_us_583e3d98e4b0ae0e7cdaca32.

51. Andrew Joseph, "After Criticism from Scientists, Congress Eases Its Pursuit
of Faster Stem Cell Therapies," STAT, November 20, 2016, https://www.statnews
.com/2016/11/30/stem-cells-cures-act/.

52. REGROW Act, https://www.congress.gov/bill/114th-congress/senate-bill
/2689.

53. Sarah Karlin-Smith, "New Stem Cell Legislation Raises Alarm," Politico,
May 2, 2016, https://www.politico.com/tipsheets/prescription-pulse/2016/05
/new-legislation-on-stem-cells-raises-alarm-214069.

54. Bipartisan Policy Center, "Advancing Regenerative Cellular Therapy:
Medical Innovation for Healthier Americans," https://bipartisanpolicy.org/events
/advancing-regenerative-cellular-therapies/.

55. Michael J. Fox Foundation for Parkinson's Disease, "MJFF Signs Letter
Opposing the REGROW Act," Foxfeed Blog, May 21, 2016, https://www
.michaeljfox.org/foundation/news-detail.php?mjff-signs-letter-opposing-the
-regrow-act.

56. Alliance for Regenerative Medicine, https://alliancerm.org/sites/default
/files/ARMSenatorKirk_REGROWActletter_March2016_.pdf.

57. International Society for Stem Cell Research, "ISSCR Opposes REGROW
Act," September 15, 2016, http://www.isscr.org/professional-resources/news
-publicationsss/isscr-news-articles/article-listing/2016/09/15/isscr-opposes
-the-regrow-act.

58. 21st Century Cures Act, http://docs.house.gov/billsthisweek/20161128
/CPRT-114-HPRT-RU00-SAHR34.pdf., 180.

59. Sarah Karlin-Smith, "New Stem Cell Legislation Raises Alarm."

60. Zachary Brennan, "Trump to Pharma CEOs: 75% to 80% of FDA Regulations
Will be Eliminated," RAPS, Regulatory Affairs Professional Society, January 31, 2017,
https://www.raps.org/news-articles/news-articles/2017/1/trump-to-pharma
-ceos–75-to–80-of-fda-regulations-will-be-eliminated.

61. Katie Thomas, "Trump's F.D.A. Pick Could Undo Decades of Drug Safeguards," *New York Times*, February 5, 2017, https://www.nytimes.com/2017/02/05
/health/with-fda-vacancy-trump-sees-chance-to-speed-drugs-to-the-market
.html.

62. Laurie McGinley and Carolyn Y. Johnson, "Trump to Select Scott Gottlieb,
a Physician with Deep Drug Industry Ties, to Run the FDA," March 10, 2017,
https://www.washingtonpost.com/news/to-your-health/wp/2017/03/10
/trump-selects-scott-gottlieb-a-physician-with-deep-drug-industry-ties-to-run
-the-fda/?utm_term=.72e452e90b75.

63. Scott Gottlieb and Coleen Klasmeier, "The FDA Wants to Regulate Your Cells," AEI.org, August 8, 2012, http://www.aei.org/article/health/the-fda-wants-to-regulate-your-cells/.

64. Food & Drug Administration, "Statement from FDA Commissioner Scott Gottlieb, MD on the FDA's New Policy Steps and Enforcement Efforts to Ensure Proper Oversight of Stem Cell Therapies and Regenerative Medicine," August 28, 2017, https://www.fda.gov/NewsEvents/Newsroom/PressAnnouncements/ucm573443.htm.

65. Ibid.

66. Ibid.

67. Food & Drug Administration, Warning Letter, US Stem Cell Clinic, LLC 8/24/17, August 2017, https://www.fda.gov/ICECI/EnforcementActions/Warning Letters/2017/ucm573187.htm.

68. Food & Drug Administration, FDA News Release, "FDA Acts to Remove Unproven, Potentially Harmful Treatment Used in 'Stem Cell' Centers Targeting Vulnerable Patients," August 28, 2017, https://www.fda.gov/NewsEvents/Newsroom/PressAnnouncements/ucm573427.htm.

69. Food & Drug Administration, News Release, "FDA Announces Comprehensive Regenerative Medicine Policy Framework," November 15, 2017, https://www.fda.gov/NewsEvents/Newsroom/PressAnnouncements/ucm585345.htm.

70. Food & Drug Administration, "Regulatory Considerations for Human Cells, Tissues, and Cellular and Tissue-Based Products: Minimal Manipulation and Homologous Use," Guidance for Industry and Food and Drug Administration Staff, November 2017 (Corrected December 2017), https://www.fda.gov/downloads/BiologicsBloodVaccines/GuidanceComplianceRegulatoryInformation/Guidances/CellularandGeneTherapy/UCM585403.pdf.

71. Ibid., 11.

72. Ibid., 13.

73. Ibid.

74. Food & Drug Administration, "FDA Announces Comprehensive Regenerative Medicine Policy Framework."

75. Leigh Turner and Paul Knoepfler, "Selling Stem Cells in the USA: Assessing the Direct-to-Consumer Industry," *Cell Stem Cell* 19, no. 2 (2016): 154–57.

76. Zachary Brennan, "FDA Unveils New Regenerative Medicine Framework," Regulatory Focus, November 16, 2017, http://raps.org/Regulatory-Focus/News/2017/11/16/28900/FDA-Unveils-New-Regenerative-Medicine-Framework/.

Chapter 8

1. Daniel Carpenter, *Reputation and Power: Organizational Image and Pharmaceutical Regulation at the FDA* (Princeton University Press, 2014).

2. Hoover Institution, "Take It to the Limits: Milton Friedman on Libertarianism," Uncommon Knowledge, 2010, https://www.hoover.org/research/take-it-limits-milton-friedman-libertarianism.

3. 21st Century Cures Act, Public Law 114-255, December 13, 2016, 1096.

4. Archibald Thomas, "They Just Know: The Epistemological Politics of 'Evidence-Based' Nonformal Education," *Evaluation and Program Planning* 48 (2015): 137–48; Alex Faulkner, *Medical Technology into Healthcare and Society: A Sociology of Devices, Innovation, and Governance* (Basingstoke, England: Palgrave MacMillan, 2009); Courtney Davis and John Abraham, "Desperately Seeking Cancer Drugs: Explaining the Emergence and Outcomes of Accelerated Pharmaceutical Regulation," *Sociology of Health and Illness* 3, no. 5 (2011): 731–47; Julie Guthman and Sandy Brown, "Whose Life Counts Biopolitics and the 'Bright Line' of Chloropicrin Mitigation in California's Strawberry Industry," *Science, Technology & Human Values* (2015): 1–22.

5. T. F. Gieryn, *Cultural Boundaries of Science: Credibility on the Line* (Chicago: University of Chicago Press, 1999).

6. Guthman and Brown, "Whose Life Counts: Biopolitics and the 'Bright Line' of Chloropicrin Mitigation in California's Strawberry Industry"; Pascale Lehoux and Stuart Blume, "Technology Assessment and the Sociopolitics of Health Technologies," *Journal of Health Politics, Policy, and Law* 25, no 6 (200): 1083–1120; M. A. Rodwin, "The Politics of Evidence-Based Medicine," *Journal of Health Politics, Policy, and Law* 26, no. 2 (2011): 438–46; Miriam Solomon, *Making Medical Knowledge* (Oxford: Oxford University Press, 2015).

7. Toby Bolson, James N. Druckman, and Fay Lomax Cook, "How Frames Can Undermine Support for Scientific Adaptations: Politicization and the Status-Quo Bias," *Public Opinion Quarterly* 78, no. 1 (2014): 1–26; I. De Melo-Martin and K. Intemann, "Interpreting Evidence: Why Values Can Matter as Much as Science," *Perspectives in Biology and Medicine* 55, no. 1 (2012): 59–70; Rosalind Edwards, Val Gillies, and Nicola Horsley, "Early Intervention and Evidence-Based Policy and Practice: Framing and Taming," *Social Policy & Society* (2015); 1–10; Narcyz Ghinea, et al., "Ethics & Evidence in Medical Debates: The Case of Recombinant Activated Factor VII," *Hastings Center Report* 44, no. 2 (2014): 38–45; J. C. Peterson and G. E. Markle, "Politics and Science in the Laetrile Controversy," *Social Studies of Science* 9 (1979): 139–66.

8. Stephen Epstein, *AIDS, Activism, and the Politics of Knowledge* (Berkeley: University of California Press, 1996); R. A. Rettig, P. D. Jacobson, and C. M. Farquhar, *False Hope: Bone Marrow Transplantation for Breast Cancer* (New York: Oxford University Press, 2007).

9. T. Baldwin, et al., *Novel Neurotechnologies: Intervening in the Brain* (London: Nuffield Council on Bioethics, 2013).

10. Charles E. Lindblom, *Politics and Markets* (New York: Basic Books, 1977).

11. Berman Elizabeth Popp, "Not Just Neoliberalism: Economization in U.S. Science and Technology Policy," *Science, Technology & Human Values* 39, no. 3 (2014): 397–431.

12. J. Patrick Woolley, "Kaufman's Debt to Kant: The Epistemological Importance of the Structure of the World Which Environs Us," *Zygon®* 48, no. 3 (2013): 544–64.

13. M. A. Rodwin, "The Politics of Evidence-Based Medicine," *Journal of Health Politics, Policy, and Law* 26, no. 2 (2011): 438–46.

14. Douglas Heather, "Politics and Science: Untangling Values, Ideologies, and Reasons," *Annals of the American Academy of Political and Social Science* 658 (2015): 296–306.

15. Sara A. Binder, *Stalemate: Causes and Consequences of Legislative Gridlock* (Washington, D.C.: Brookings Institution, 2003); Denise F. Lillvis, Anna Kirkland, and Anna Frick, "Power and Persuasion in the Vaccine Debates: An Analysis of Political Efforts and Outcomes in the United States, 1998–2012," *Milbank Quarterly* 92, no. 3 (2014): 475–508.

16. Eric C. Nisbet, Kathryn E. Cooper, and Garrett R. Kelly, "The Partisan Brain: How Dissonant Science Messages Lead Conservatives and Liberals to (Dis)trust Science," *The ANNALS of the American Academy of Political and Social Science* 658, no. 1 (2015): 36–66; Matthew Nisbet and Ezra M. Markowitz, "Understanding Public Opinion in Debates Over Biomedical Research: Looking Beyond Political Partisanship to Focus on Beliefs About Science and Society," *PloS One* 9, no 2 (2014): e88473.

17. Toby Bolsen, James N. Druckman, and Fay Lomax Cook, "How Frames Can Undermine Support for Scientific Adaptations: Politicization and the Status-Quo Bias," *Public Opinion Quarterly* 78, no. 1 (2014): 1–26; Douglas Heather, "Politics and Science: Untangling Values, Ideologies and Reasons," *Annals of the American Academy of Political and Social Science* 658 (2015): 296–306.

18. Aaron M. McCright, et al., "The Influence of Political Ideology on Trust in Science," *Environmental Research Letters* 8, no. 4 (2013): 044029.

19. Ed Silverman, "Avastin & FDA Were Both on Trial: Dan Explains," Pharmalot, June 20, 2011, http://pharmalot.com/2011/06/avastin-fda-were-both-on -trial-carpenter-explains/

20. Murial R. Gillick, "The Technological Imperative and the Battle for the Hearts of America," *Perspectives in Biology and Medicine* 50, no. 2 (2007): 276–94.

21. Rettig, et al., *False Hope: Bone Marrow Transplantation for Breast Cancer.*

22. Christopher Jewell and Lisa Bero, "Public Participation and Claimsmaking: Evidence Utilization and Divergent Policy Frames in California's Ergonomics Rulemaking," *Journal of Public Administration Research and Theory* 17, no. 4 (2007):625–50.

23. D. Schön and M. Rein, *Frame Reflection: Toward the Resolution of Intractable Policy Controversies* (New York: Basic Books, 1994).

24. Liesbet van Zoonen, "I-pistemology: Changing Truth Claims in Popular and Political Culture," *European Journal of Communication* 27, no. 1 (2012): 65–67.

25. Rachel Grob, *Testing Baby: The Transformation of Newborn Screening, Parenting, and Policymaking* (Rutgers University Press, 2011); Michael K. Gusmano; "FDA Decisions and Public Deliberation: Challenges and Opportunities," *Public Administration Review* 73, no. S1 (2013): S115–S126.

26. J. D. Chambers, et al., "Medicare Is Scrutinizing Evidence More Tightly for National Coverage Determinations," *Health Affairs* 34, no. 2: (2015): 253–60; J. D. Chambers, P. J. Neumann, and M. J. Buxton, "Does Medicare Have an

Implicit Cost-Effectiveness Threshold?" *Medical Decision Making* 30 (2010): E14–E27; P. J. Neumann, A. B. Rosen, and M. C. Weinstein, "Medicare and Cost-Effectiveness Analysis," *New England Journal of Medicine* 353, no. 14 (2005): 1516–22.

27. Peter J. Neumann and Sean R. Tunis, "Medicare and Medical Technology—The Growing Demand for Relevant Outcomes," *New England Journal of Medicine* 362, no. 5 (2010): 377–79.

28. C. Sorenson, M. K. Gusmano, and A. Oliver, "The Politics of Comparative Effectiveness Research: Lessons from Recent History," *Journal of Health Politics, Policy, and Law* 3, no. 1 (2014): 139–69.

29. Emma Court, "At $300,000 a Year, Sarepta's New Drug Is Considered a Steal," *Market Watch*, September 21, 2016, https://www.marketwatch.com/story/at-300000-a-year-sareptas-new-drug-is-considered-a-steal-2016-09-20; Katie Thomas, "Insurers Battle Families Over Costly Drug for Fatal Disease," *New York Times*, June 22, 2017, https://www.nytimes.com/2017/06/22/health/duchenne-muscular-dystrophy-drug-exondys-51.html.

30. Thomas, "Insurers Battle Families Over Costly Drug for Fatal Disease."

31. Karen J. Maschke, Michael K. Gusmano, and Mildred Z. Solomon, "Breakthrough Cancer Treatments Raise Difficult Questions," *Health Affairs* 36, no. 10 (2017): 1698–1700.

32. Liz Szabo, "Breakthrough Cancer Drug Could Be Astronomical in Price," *USA Today*, August 22, 2017, https://www.usatoday.com/story/news/2017/08/22/breakthrough-cancer-drug-astronomical-price/589442001/.

33. Michael Ollove, "Are States Obligated to Provide Expensive Hepatitis C Drugs?" *The PEW Charitable Trusts*, February 9, 2016, http://www.pewtrusts.org/en/research-and-analysis/blogs/stateline/2016/02/09/are-states-obligated-to-provide-expensive-hepatitis-c-drugs.

34. Szabo, "Breakthrough Cancer Drug Could Be Astronomical in Price."

35. Ibid.

36. Ibid.

37. Arlene Weintraub, "How to Cover Novartis' $475K CAR-T Drug Kymriah? A 'New Payment Model' Is the Only Way, Express Scripts Says," FiercePharma, September 22, 2017, https://www.fiercepharma.com/financials/car-t-and-other-gene-therapies-need-new-payment-model-says-express-scripts.

38. Szabo, "Breakthrough Cancer Drug Could Be Astronomical in Price,"

39. Liz Szabo, "Cascade of Costs Could Push New Gene Therapy Above $1 Million per Patient," *Kaiser Health News*, October 17, 2017, https://khn.org/news/cascade-of-costs-could-push-new-gene-therapy-above-1-million-per-patient/.

40. Ibid.

41. Mildred Z. Solomon, Michael K. Gusmano, and Karen J. Maschke, "The Ethical Imperative and Moral Challenges of Engaging Patients and the Public with Evidence. *Health Affairs* 35 (2015): 4583–89.

42. Paul Kleutghen, et al., "Drugs Don't Work if People Can't Afford Them: The High Price of Tisagenlecleucel," *Health Affairs Blog*, February 8, 2018, https://www.healthaffairs.org/do/10.1377/hblog20180205.292531/full/.

43. D. J. Fiorino, "Citizen Participation and Environmental Risk: A Survey of Institutional Mechanisms," *Science, Technology & Human Values* 15, no. 2 (1990): 226–43.

44. National Research Council, "Public Engagement on Genetically Modified Organisms: When Science and Citizens Connect: Workshop Summary" (Washington, D.C.: National Academies Press, 2015).

45. Gregory E. Kaebnick and Michael K. Gusmano, "CBA and Precaution: Policy-Making about Emerging Technologies," *Hastings Center Report* 48, no. 1 (2018): S88–S96.

46. Ibid.

47. G. Rowe and L. J. Frewer, "A Typology of Public Engagement Mechanisms," *Science, Technology & Human Values* 30, no. 2 (2005): 25–90.

48. Carol Pateman, *Participation and Democratic Theory* (Cambridge: University Press, 1970).

49. Stephanie Solomon and Julia Abelson, "Why and When Should We Use Public Deliberation?" *Hastings Center Report* 42, no. 2 (2012): 17–20.

50. D. Menon and T. Stafinski, "Engaging the Public in Priority-Setting for Health Technology Assessment: Findings from a Citizens' Jury," *Health Expectations* 11 (2008): 282–93.

51. F. Merali Chafe, et al., "Does the Public Think it Is Reasonable to Wait for More Evidence before Funding Innovative Health Technologies? The Case of PET Screening in Ontario," *International Journal of Technology Assessment in Health Care* 26 (2010): 192–97.

52. Anthony J. Culyer, "Involving Stakeholders in Healthcare Decisions—The Experience of the National Institute for Clinical Excellence (NICE) in England and Wales," *Healthcare Quarterly* 8, no. 3 (2005): 54–58.

53. USPSTF. https://www.uspreventiveservicestaskforce.org/.

54. Medical Device Innovation Consortium, "Medical Device Innovation Consortium (MDIC) Patient-Centered Benefit-Risk Project Report," n.d., http://mdic.org/wp-content/uploads/2015/05/MDIC_Summary_Report_SinglePage_5.7.15.pdf.

55. Ibid., 6.

56. Food & Drug Administration, Patient Engagement Advisory Committee, https://www.fda.gov/AdvisoryCommittees/CommitteesMeetingMaterials/PatientEngagementAdvisoryCommittee/default.htm, 5707.

57. Ibid.

58. 21st Century Cures Act. Public Law 114-255-Dec. 13, 2016: 133

59. Food & Drug Administration, FDA Statement, "Statement by FDA Commissioner Scott Gottlieb, MD, on New Steps by FDA to Advance Patient Engagement in the Agency's Regulatory Work," October 11, 2017, https://www.fda.gov/NewsEvents/Newsroom/PressAnnouncements/ucm579842.htm.

60. Ibid., 5.

61. Michael K. Gusmano, "FDA Decisions and Public Deliberation: Challenges and Opportunities," *Public Administration Review* 73, no. S1 (2013): S115–S126; Grob, *Testing Baby: The Transformation of Newborn Screening, Parenting, and Policymaking.*

62. Food & Drug Administration, FDA Statement, "FDA Commissioner Scott Gottlieb, MD, on New Steps FDA Is Taking to Enhance Transparency of Clinical Trial Information to Support Innovation and Scientific Inquiry Related to New Drugs," January 16, 2018, https://www.fda.gov/NewsEvents/Newsroom/Press Announcements/ucm592566.htm.

63. Ibid., 2.

64. Daniel Carpenter, *Reputation and Power: Organizational Image and Pharmaceutical Regulation at the FDA* (Princeton University Press, 2014); Daniel Carpenter, "Strengthen and Stabilize the FDA," *Nature* 485: 169–70.

65. Office of Inspector General, "Local Coverage Determinations Create Inconsistency in Medicare Coverage."

66. J. R. Trosman, S. L. Van Bebber, and K. A. Phillips, "Coverage Policy Development for Personalized Medicine: Private Payer Perspectives on Developing Policy for the 21-Gene Assay," *Journal of Oncology Practice* 6, no. 5 (2010): 238–42.

67. M. D. Graf, et al., "Genetic Testing Insurance Coverage Trends: A Review of Publicly Available Policies from the Largest U.S. Payers," *Personalized Medicine* 10, no. 3 (2013): 235–43; A. Hresko and S. B. Haga, "Insurance Coverage Policies for Personalized Medicine," *Journal of Personalized Medicine* 2, no. 4 (2012): 201–16; J. R. Trosman, et al., "Challenges of Coverage Policy Development for Next-Generation Tumor Sequencing Panels: Experts and Payers Weigh In," *Journal of the National Comprehensive Cancer Network* 13, no. 3 (2015): 312–18; J. R. Trosman, et al., "What Do Providers, Payers, and Patients Need from Comparative Effectiveness Research on Diagnostics? The Case of HER2/Neu Testing in Breast Cancer," *Journal of Comparative Effectiveness Research* 2, no. 4 (2013): 461–77; J. R. Trosman, S. L. Van Bebber, and K. A. Phillips, "Health Technology Assessment and Private Payers' Coverage of Personalized Medicine," *Journal of Oncology Practice* 7, no. 3S (2011): 18s–24s; Trosman, et al., "Coverage Policy Development for Personalized Medicine: Private Payer Perspectives on Developing Policy for the 21-Gene Assay."

Bibliography

Abraham, John and Rachel Ballinger. "The Neoliberal Regulatory State, Industry Interests, and the Ideological Penetration of Scientific Knowledge: Deconstructing the Redefinition of Carcinogens in Pharmaceuticals." *Science, Technology & Human Values* 37, no. 5 (2012): 443–77.

Adams, Samuel Hopkins. *The Great American Fraud: Articles on the Nostrum Evil and Quacks, in Two Series.* Reprinted by *Collier's Weekly,* 4th edition. New York: P.F. Collier & Son, 1911.

Aebi, Stefan, Shari Gelber, Stewart J. Anderson, István Láng, André Robidoux, Miguel Martín, Johan W. R. Nortier, Alexander H. G. Paterson, Mothaffar F. Rimawi, José Manuel Baena Cañada, Beat Thürlimann, Elizabeth Murray, Eleftherios P. Mamounas, Charles E. Geyer, Jr., Karen N. Price, Alan S. Coates, Richard D. Gelber, Priya Rastogi, Norman Wolmark, and Irene L. Wapnir. "Chemotherapy for Isolated Locoregional Recurrence of Breast Cancer: The CALOR Randomised Trial." *Lancet Oncology* 15, no. 2 (2014): 156–63.

Albert, Marilyn S., Steven T. DeKosky, Dennis Dickson, Bruno Dubois, Howard H. Feldman, Nick C. Fox, Anthony Gamst, David M. Holtzman, William J. Jagust, Ronald C. Petersen, Peter J. Snyder, Maria C. Carrillo, Bill Thies, and Creighton H. Phelps. "The Diagnosis of Mild Cognitive Impairment Due to Alzheimer's Disease: Recommendations from the National Institute on Aging-Alzheimer's Association Workgroups on Diagnostic Guidelines for Alzheimer's Disease." *Alzheimer's & Dementia* 7, no. 3 (2011): 270–79.

Alliance for Regenerative Medicine. "Technologies." https://alliancerm.org/technologies/; accessed May 22, 2018.

ALZ Forum. "Alzheimer's Community Mobilizes to Show Benefits of Amyloid Scans." October 11, 2013. https://www.alzforum.org/news/community-news/alzheimers-community-mobilizes-show-benefits-amyloid-scans; accessed May 22, 2018.

ALZ Forum. "Coverage Denial for Amyloid Scans Riles Alzheimer's Community." July 25, 2013. http://www.alzforum.org/news/conference-coverage/coverage-denial-amyloid-scans-riles-alzheimers-community; accessed May 22, 2018.

Alzheimer's Association. "Alzheimer's Disease Facts and Figures." 2015. https://www.alz.org/facts/downloads/facts_figures_2015.pdf; accessed May 22, 2018.

Alzheimer's Association. "What Is Dementia?" https://www.alz.org/what-is-dementia.asp; accessed May 22, 2018.

American Cancer Society. *Breast Cancer Facts and Figures, 2017–2018*. https://www.cancer.org/content/dam/cancer-org/research/cancer-facts-and-statistics/breast-cancer-facts-and-figures/breast-cancer-facts-and-figures-2017-2018.pdf; accessed May 22, 2018.

American Cancer Society. "NIH to Fund Study of Breast Cancer in Black Women." American Cancer Society, 2016, https://www.cancer.org/latest-news/nih-to-fund-study-of-breast-cancer-in-black-women.html; accessed May 22, 2018.

Anderson, Gerard F., B. K. Frogner, and Uwe Reinhardt. "Health Spending in OECD Countries in 2004: An Update." *Health Affairs* 26, no. 5 (2007): 1481–89.

Andrews, Michelle. "FDA's Approval of a Cheaper Drug for Hepatitis C Will Likely Expand Treatment." *NPR*. October 4, 2017. https://www.npr.org/sections/health-shots/2017/10/04/555156577/fdas-approval-of-a-cheaper-drug-for-hepatitis-c-will-likely-expand-treatment; accessed May 22, 2018.

Angell, Marcia. *The Truth About Drug Companies: How They Deceive Us and What to Do About It*. New York: Random House, 2005.

Arno, Peter and Michael H. Davis. "At Issue: Should Medicare Be Allowed to Negotiate Drug Prices?" *CQ Researcher* 26, no. 20 (2016): 473.

Arno, Peter S. and Michael H. Davis. "The New Face of US Health Care: $1,000 per Pill." *Truthout*. December 23, 2014. http://www.truth-out.org/opinion/item/28171-the-new-face-of-us-health-care-1-000-per-pill; accessed May 22, 2018.

Ashcroft, Richard E. "Current Epistemological Problems in Evidence-Based Medicine." *Journal of Medical Ethics* 30 (2004): 131–35.

Ashley, J. R. and Cecine N. Nguyen. "A Comparison of Cancer Burden and Research Spending Reveals Discrepancies in the Distribution of Research Funding." *BMC Public Health* 12 (2012): 526.

Avorn, Jerry and Aaron S. Kesselheim. "The 21st Century Cures Act—Will It Take Us Back in Time?" *New England Journal of Medicine* 372, no. 26 (2015): 2473–75.

Backus, Lisa I., Derek B. Boothroyd, Barbara R. Phillips, Pamela Belperio, James Halloran, and Larry A. Mole. "A Sustained Virologic Response Reduces Risk of All-Cause Mortality in Patients with Hepatitis C." *Clinical Gastroenterology and Hepatology* 9 (2011): 509–16.

Bagley, Nicholas. "Who Says PCORI Can't Do Cost Effectiveness?" The Incidental Economists: A Health Services Research Blog. October 14, 2013. http://theincidentaleconomist.com/wordpress/who-says-pcori-cant-do-cost-effectiveness/; accessed May 22, 2018.

Baines, Cornelia J. "Rational and Irrational Issues in Breast Cancer Screening." *Cancers* 3, no. 1 (2011): 252–66.

Baldwin T., M. Fitzgerald, J. Kitzinger, G. Laurie, J. Price, N. Rose, S. Rose, I. Singh, V. Walsh, and K. Warwick. *Novel Neurotechnologies: Intervening in the Brain.* London: Nuffield Council on Bioethics, 2013.

Ball, Robert M. "What Medicare's Architects Had in Mind." *Health Affairs* 14, no. 4 (1995): 62–72.

Baptista, Pedro M. and Anthony Atala. "Regenerative Medicine: The Hurdles and Hopes." In *Translating Regenerative Medicine to the Clinic*, edited by Jeffrey Laurence, Pedro M. Baptista and Anthony Atala, 3–7. Amsterdam: Elsevier, 2016.

Beckman, Adam, Alyssa Bilinski, Ryan Boyko, George M. Camp, A. T. Wall, Joseph K. Lim, Emily A. Wang, R. Douglas Bruce, and Gregg S. Gonsalves. "New Hepatitis C Drugs are Very Costly and Unavailable to Many State Prisoners." *Health Affairs* 35, no. 10 (2017): 1893–1901.

Beil, Laura. "Stem Cell Treatments Overtake Science." *New York Times.* September 9, 2013. http://www.nytimes.com/2013/09/10/health/stem-cell-treatments-overtake-science.html; accessed May 22, 2018.

Béland, Daniel. "Ideas and Social Policy: An Institutionalist Perspective." *Social Policy & Administration* 39, no 1 (2005): 1–18.

Béland, Daniel. "Reconsidering Policy Feedback: How Policies Affect Politics." *Administration & Policy* 2010, 42(5): 568–90.

Berfield, Susan. "Stem Cell Showdown: Celltex versus the FDA." *Bloomberg Businessweek.* January 3, 2013. http://www.businessweek.com/articles/2013-01-03/stem-cell-showdown-celltex-vs-dot-the-fda; accessed May 22, 2018.

Bergthold, Linda A. "Medical Necessity: Do We Need It?" *Health Affairs* 14, no. 4 (1995): 180–90.

Berkman, Lisa F., Ichiro Kawachi, and Maria Glymour, eds. *Social Epidemiology*, 2nd edition. Oxford: Oxford University Press, 2014.

Berkowitz, Edward. "History of Health Services Research Project Interview with Barbara Starfield." U.S. National Library of Medicine, 2003. https://www.nlm.nih.gov/hmd/nichsr/starfield.html; accessed May 22, 2018.

Berwick, Donald. "A User's Manual for the IOM's 'Quality Chasm' Report." *Health Affairs* 21, no. 3 (2002): 80–90.

Binder, Sara A. *Stalemate: Causes and Consequences of Legislative Gridlock.* Washington, D.C.: Brookings Institution, 2003.

Bipartisan Policy Center. "Advancing Regenerative Cellular Therapy: Medical Innovation for Healthier Americans." https://bipartisanpolicy.org/events/advancing-regenerative-cellular-therapies/; accessed May 22, 2018.

Birkland, Thomas A. "Focusing Events, Mobilization, and Agenda Setting." *Journal of Public Policy* 18, no. 1 (1998): 53–74.

Blake, Valarie. "The Terminally Ill, Access to Investigational Drugs, and FDA Rules." *AMA Journal of Ethics* 15, no. 8 (2013): 687–91.

Bleyer, Archie and H. Gilbert Welch. "Effect of Three Decades of Screening Mammography on Breast-Cancer Incidence." *New England Journal of Medicine* 367, no. 21 (2012): 1998–2005.

Blumenthal, David and Charles M. Kilo. "A Report Card on Continuous Quality Improvement." *The Milbank Quarterly* 76, no. 4 (1998): 625–48.

Blumenthal, David, Karen Davis, and Stuart Guterman. "Medicare at 50— Origins and Evolution." *New England Journal of Medicine* 372, no. 7 (2015): 671–77.

Bolson, Toby, James N. Druckman, and Fay Lomax Cook. "How Frames Can Undermine Support for Scientific Adaptations: Politicization and the Status-Quo Bias." *Public Opinion Quarterly* 78, no. 1 (2014): 1–26.

Booth, Christopher M. and Elizabeth A. Eisenhauer. "Progression-Free Survival: Meaningful or Simply Measurable?" *Journal of Clinical Oncology* 30, no. 10 (2012): 1030–33.

Bothwell, Laura E., Jeremy A. Greene, Scott H. Podolsky, and David S. Jones. "Assessing the Gold Standard—Lessons from the History of RCTs." *New England Journal of Medicine* 374 (2016): 2175–81.

Braun, Susan. "The History of Breast Cancer Advocacy." *The Breast Journal* 9, no. s2 (2003): S101–S103.

Brennan, Zachary. "FDA Unveils New Regenerative Medicine Framework." Regulatory Focus. November 16, 2017. http://raps.org/Regulatory-Focus /News/2017/11/16/28900/FDA-Unveils-New-Regenerative-Medicine -Framework/; accessed May 22, 2018.

Brennan, Zachary. "Trump to Pharma CEOs: 75% to 80% of FDA Regulations Will Be Eliminated." RAPS, Regulatory Affairs Professional Society. January 31, 2017. https://www.raps.org/news-articles/news-articles/2017/1 /trump-to-pharma-ceos-75-to-80-of-fda-regulations-will-be-eliminated; accessed May 22, 2018.

Brook, Robert H. "Practice Guidelines and Practicing Medicine: Are They Compatible?" *Journal of the American Medical Association* 262 (1989): 3027–30.

Brook, Robert H., Mark R. Chassin, and Arlene Fink. "A Method for Detailed Assessment of the Appropriateness of Medical Technologies." *International Journal Technology Assessment in Health Care* 2 (1986): 53–63.

Brook, Robert H., Kathleen Lohr, Mark Chassin, Jacqueline Kosecoff, Arlene Fink, and David Solomon. "Geographic Variations in the Use of Services: Do They Have Any Clinical Significance?" *Health Affairs* 3, no. 2 (1984): 63–73.

Brook, Robert H., K. N. Williams, and J. E. Rolph. "Controlling the Use and Cost of Medical Services: The New Mexico Experimental Medical Care Review Organization—A Four-Year Case Study." *Medical Care* 16, no. 9, Suppl. (1978): 1–76.

Brower, Vicki. "The Squeaky Wheel Gets the Grease." *EMBO Reports* 6, no. 11 (2005): 1014–17.

Bulik, Beth Snyder. "Gilead Pushes Hep C Testing in Baby Boomers as its Blockbusters Plummet." *FiercePharma.* February 22, 2017. https://www

.fiercepharma.com/marketing/baby-boomers-targeted-gilead-hepatitis-c
-awareness-campaign-even-as-drug-s-fortunes-drop; accessed May
22, 2018.

Burstow, Nicholas J., Zameer Mohamed, Asmaa I. Gomaa, Mark W. Sonderup, Nicola A. Cook, Imam Waked, C. Wendy Spearman, and Simon D. Taylor-Robinson. "Hepatitis C Treatment: Where Are We Now?" *International Journal of General Medicine* 10 (2017): 39–52.

Burton, Thomas M. and Jennifer Corbett Dooren. "Key FDA Approval Yanked for Avastin." *Wall Street Journal.* November 19, 2011. https://www.wsj.com/articles/SB10001424052970203699404577046041941288780; accessed May 22, 2018.

Callahan, Daniel. "Controlling Costs: Do as Business Does." *Health Care Cost Monitor.* January 29, 2009.

Callahan, Daniel. *Taming the Beloved Beast: How Medical Technology Is Ruining Our Health System.* Oxford: Oxford University Press, 2009.

Callahan, Daniel. *What Kind of Life: The Limits of Medical Progress.* New York: Simon and Schuster, 1990.

Calonge, N, D. B. Petitti, T. G. DeWitt, A. J. Dietrich, K. D. Gregory, D. Grossman, G. Isham, M. L. LeFevre, R. M. Leipzig, L. N. Marion, B. Melnyk, V. A. Moyer, J. K. Ocke, G. F. Sawaya, J. S. Schwartz, and T. Wilt. "Screening for Breast Cancer: U.S. Preventive Services Task Force Recommendation Statement." *Annals of Internal Medicine* 151, no. 10 (2009): 716–26.

Campbell, John L. "Ideas, Politics, and Public Policy." *Annual Review of Sociology* 28 (2002): 21–38.

Cannon, Michael F. "A Better Way to Generate and Use Comparative-Effectiveness Research." *Policy Analysis* 632 (2009): 1–21.

Carnahan, Sandra J. "Medicare's Coverage with Study Participation Policy: Clinical Trials or Tribulations." *Yale Journal of Health Policy Law & Ethics* 7, no. 2 (2007): 229–72.

Carpenter, Daniel. *Reputation and Power: Organizational Image and Pharmaceutical Regulation at the FDA.* Princeton, NJ: Princeton University Press, 2014.

Carpenter, Daniel. "Strengthen and Stabilize the FDA." *Nature* 485 (2012): 169–70.

Casamayou, Maureen Hogan. "The Breast Cancer Wars: Hope, Fear, and the Pursuit of a Cure in Twentieth-Century America." *Journal of Health Politics, Policy, and Law* 27, no. 6 (2002): 1037–39.

Casamayou, Maureen Hogan. *The Politics of Breast Cancer.* Washington, D.C.: Georgetown University Press, 2001.

Cavers, David F. "The Food, Drug, and Cosmetic Act of 1938: Its Legislative History and Its Substantive Provisions." *Law and Contemporary Problems* 6, no. 1 (1939): 2–42.

Centers for Disease Control and Prevention. "Hepatitis C FAQs for the Public." https://www.cdc.gov/hepatitis/hcv/cfaq.htm#cFAQ35; accessed May 22, 2018.

Chafe, Roger, Farhan Merali, Andreas Laupacis, Wendy Levinson, and Doug Martin. "Does the Public Think It Is Reasonable to Wait for More Evidence before Funding Innovative Health Technologies? The Case of PET Screening in Ontario." *International Journal of Technology Assessment in Health Care* 26 (2010): 192–97.

Chak, E. W., S. Sarkar, and C. Bowlus. "Improving Healthcare Systems to Reduce Healthcare Disparities in Viral Hepatitis." *Digestive Diseases and Sciences* 61, no. 10 (2016): 2776–83.

Chambers, James D., Matthew D. Chenoweth, Michael J. Cangelosi, Junhee Pyo, Joshua T. Cohen, and Peter J. Neumann. "Medicare Is Scrutinizing Evidence More Tightly for National Coverage Determinations." *Health Affairs* 34, no. 2 (2015): 253–60.

Chambers, James D., Matthew D. Chenoweth, Junhee Pyo, Michael J. Cangelosi, and Peter J. Neumann. "Changing Face of Medicare's National Coverage Determinations for Technology." *International Journal of Technology Assessment in Health Care* 31, no. 5 (2016): 1–8.

Chambers, James D., K. E. May, and P. J. Neumann. "Medicare Covers the Majority of FDA-Approved Devices and Part B Drugs, but Restrictions and Discrepancies Remain." *Health Affairs* 32, no. 6, (2013): 1109–15.

Chambers, James D., P. J. Neumann, and M. J. Buxton. "Does Medicare Have an Implicit Cost-Effectiveness Threshold?" *Medical Decision Making* 30 (2010): E14–E27.

Charles, Amber M. "Indifference, Interruption, and Immunodeficiency: The Impact and Implications of Inadequate HIV/AIDS Care in U.S. Prisons." *Boston University Law Review* 92, no. 6 (2012): 1979–2022.

Chassin, Mark. "Variations in the Use of Medical and Surgical Services by the Medicare Population." *New England Journal of Medicine* 314, no. 5 (1986): 285–90.

Chen, H. X. and J. N. Cleck. "Adverse Effects of Anticancer Agents that Target the VEGF Pathway." *Nature Reviews Clinical Oncology* 6, no. 8 (2009): 464–77.

Chen, Liyan. "The Most Profitable Industries In 2016." *Forbes.* December 21, 2016. https://www.forbes.com/sites/liyanchen/2015/12/21/the-most -profitable-industries-in-2016/#1e6b80ab5716; accessed May 22, 2018.

Chirba, Mary Anne and Alice Noble. "Medical Malpractice, the Affordable Care Act, and State Provider Shield Laws: More Myth than Necessity?" Boston College Law School Faculty Papers, 2013.

CMS. "Beta Amyloid Positron Emission Tomography (PET) in Dementia and Neurodegenerative Disease." Medicare Evidence Development & Coverage Advisory Committee. January 30, 2013. https://www.cms.gov /medicare-coverage-database/details/medcac-meeting-details.aspx? MEDCACId=66; accessed May 22, 2018.

CMS. "Decision Memo for Beta Amyloid Positron Emission Tomography in Dementia and Neurodegenerative Disease (CAG-0431N)." September 27, 2013. https://www.cms.gov/medicare-coverage-database/details/nca -decision-memo.aspx?NCAId=265; accessed May 22, 2018.

CMS. "Medicare Program; Revised Process for Making National Determinations." *Federal Register* 78, no. 152 (August 7, 2013): 48164–69.

CMS. "What Medicare Covers." 2018. https://www.medicare.gov/what-medicare-covers/index.html; accessed May 22, 2018.

Coburn, Thomas. "Majority's Health Bill Empowers Government Task Force at Center of Mammogram Controversy." 2009. From website of Senator Tom Coburn (R-OK). http://coburn.library.okstate.edu/right_now/2009/12/senate-health-care-bill-costs-taxpayers-6-8-million-per-word.html; accessed May 22, 2018.

Cochrane Collaboration. *Cochrane Handbook for Systematic Reviews of Interventions.* Cochrane Training, GRADE Working Group. 2015. http://training.cochrane.org/handbook; accessed May 22, 2018.

Cohen, M. H., J. Gootenberg, P. Keegan, and R. Pazdur. "FDA Drug Approval Summary: Bevacizumab (Avastin) Plus Carboplatin and Paclitaxel as First-Line Treatment of Advanced/Metastatic Recurrent Nonsquamous Non-Small-Cell Lung Cancer." *Oncologist* 12, no. 6 (2007): 713–18.

Committee on Ways and Means, Subcommittee on Health, U.S. House of Representatives. *Medpac Report on Medicare Payment Policies.* Hearing, One Hundred Eighth Congress, First Session, March 6. Serial. No. 108–14 (Washington, D.C.: U.S. Government Printing Office, 2003).

Cooke, Molly, David M. Irby, William Sullivan, and Kenneth M. Ludmerer. "American Medical Education 100 Years after the Flexner Report." *New England Journal of Medicine* 355, no. 13 (2006): 1339–44.

Corbett Julia B. and Motomi Mori. "Medicine, Media, and Celebrities: News Coverage of Breast Cancer, 1960–1995." *Journalism and Mass Communication Quarterly* 76, no. 2 (1999): 229–49.

Corieri, Christina. "Everyone Deserves the Right to Try: Empowering the Terminally Ill to Take Control of Their Treatment." Goldwater Institute. February 11, 2014. https://goldwaterinstitute.org/wp-content/uploads/cms_page_media/2015/1/29/Right%20To%20Try.pdf; accessed May 22, 2018.

Cotter, Dennis. "The National Center for Health Technology: Lessons Learned." *Health Affairs Blog.* January 22, 2009. https://www.healthaffairs.org/do/10.1377/hblog20090122.000490/full/; accessed January 16, 2018.

Court, Emma. "At $300,000 a Year, Sarepta's New Drug Is Considered a Steal." *Market Watch.* September 21, 2016. https://www.marketwatch.com/story/at-300000-a-year-sareptas-new-drug-is-considered-a-steal-2016-09-20; accessed May 22, 2018.

Cruse, Julius M. "History of Medicine: The Metamorphosis of Scientific Medicine in the Ever-Present Past." *American Journal of the Medical Sciences* 318, no.3 (1999): 171–80.

Culyer, Anthony J. "Involving Stakeholders in Healthcare Decisions—The Experience of the National Institute for Clinical Excellence (NICE) in England and Wales." *Healthcare Quarterly* 8, no. 3 (2005): 54–58.

Cutler, David M. *Your Money or Your Life: Strong Medicine for America's Health Care System* New York: Oxford University Press, 2004.

Cyranoski, David B. "Celltex Makes Bold Marketing Claims Despite Significant Manufacturing Problems Found During FDA Inspection." *Health in the Global Village*. August 7, 2012.

Cyranoski, David B. "Stem Cells in Texas: Cowboy Culture." *Nature* 494, no. 7436 (2013): 166–68.

Darrow, Jonathan J., Jerry Avorn, and Aaron S. Kesselheim. "New FDA Breakthrough-Drug Category—Implications for Patients." *New England Journal of Medicine* 370, no. 13 (2014): 1252–58.

Davis, Courtney and John Abraham. "Desperately Seeking Cancer Drugs: Explaining the Emergence and Outcomes of Accelerated Pharmaceutical Regulation." *Sociology of Health and Illness* 3, no. 5 (2011): 731–47.

Davis, Michael Henry, Peter S. Arno, and Karen Bonuck. "Rare Diseases, Drug Development and AIDS: The Impact of the Orphan Drug Act." Law Faculty Articles and Essays. Cleveland State University, 1995.

De Melo-Martin, I. and K. Intemann. "Interpreting Evidence: Why Values Can Matter as Much as Science." *Perspectives in Biology and Medicine* 55, no. 1 (2012): 59–70.

den Brok, Wendie D., Caroline H. Speers, Lovedeep Gondara, Emily Baxter, Scott K. Tyldesley, Caroline A. Lohrisch. "Survival with Metastatic Breast Cancer Based on Initial Presentation, De Novo versus Relapsed." *Breast Cancer Research and Treatment* 161, no. 3 (2017): 549–56.

Dickinson, James G. "It's Time to Replace the FDA, Says Newt Gingrich." *MM&N*. May 1, 2014. https://www.mmm-online.com/legalregulatory/its-time-to-replace-the-fda-says-newt-gingrich/article/343560/; accessed May 22, 2018.

Dickson, Virgil. "Reform Update: Medicaid Programs Crafting Limits on Harvoni Usage." *Modern Healthcare*. October 21, 2014. http://www.modernhealthcare.com/article/20141021/NEWS/310219962; accessed May 22, 2018.

Donabedian, A. "Evaluating the Quality of Medical Care." *The Milbank Memorial Fund Quarterly* 44, no. 3, pt. 2 (1966): 166–203.

"Donnelly and Chairman of House Energy and Commerce Committee Discuss Bipartisan Efforts to Accelerate Medical Breakthroughs." November 16, 2015. https://www.donnelly.senate.gov/newsroom/press/donnelly-and-chairman-of-house-energy-and-commerce-committee-discuss-bipartisan-efforts-to-accelerate-medical-breakthroughs; accessed May 22, 2018.

Douglas, Heather. "Politics and Science: Untangling Values, Ideologies, and Reasons." *Annals of the American Academy of Political and Social Science* 658 (2015): 296–306.

Drabiak-Syed, Katherine. "Challenging the FDA's Authority to Regulate Autologous Adult Stem Cells for Therapeutic Use: Celltex Therapeutics' Partnership with RNL Bio, Substantial Medical Risks, and the Implications of United States v. Regenerative Sciences." *Health Matrix* 23 (2013): 493–535.

Dresser, Rebecca. *When Science Offers Salvation: Patient Advocacy and Research Ethics.* New York: Oxford University Press, 2001.

Eastman, Peggy. "NCI Adopts New Mammography Screening Guidelines for Women." *Journal of the National Cancer Institute* 89, no. 8 (1997): 538–50.

Eaton, Margaret L. and Donald Kennedy. *Innovation in Medical Technology.* Baltimore: Johns Hopkins University Press, 2009.

Edwards, Rosalind, Val Gillies, and Nicola Horsley. "Early Intervention and Evidence-Based Policy and Practice: Framing and Taming." *Social Policy & Society* 15, no. 1 (2015): 1–10.

Egan, Robert L. "Fifty-Three Cases of Carcinoma of the Breast: Occult Until Mammography." *American Journal of Roentgenology* 88 (1962): 1095–1101.

Eisenberg, M. and D. Zarin. "Health Technology Assessment in the United States. Past, Present, and Future." *International Journal of Technology Assessment in Health Care* 18, no. 2 (2002): 192–98.

Elbel, Brian and Mark Schlesinger. "Responsive Consumerism: Empowerment in Markets for Health Plans." *The Milbank Quarterly* 87, no. 3 (2009): 633–82.

Elshaug, Adam G., Janet E. Hiller, Sean R. Tunis, and John R. Moss. "Challenges in Australian Policy Processes for Disinvestment from Existing, Ineffective Health Care Practices." *Australia and New Zealand Health Policy* 4 (2007): 23.

Epstein, Andrew J. "Do Cardiac Surgery Report Cards Reduce Mortality? Assessing the Evidence." *Medical Care Research and Review* 63, no. 4 (2006): 403–26.

Epstein, Steven. *Impure Science: AIDS, Activism, and the Politics of Knowledge.* Berkeley: University of California Press, 1996.

Ernster, Virginia L. "Mammography Screening for Women Aged 40 through 499—A Guidelines Saga and a Clarion Call for Informed Decision Making." *American Journal of Public Health* 87, no. 7 (1997): 1103–06.

Faulkner, Alex. *Medical Technology into Healthcare and Society.* London: Palgrave, 2009.

Federal Food, Drug, and Cosmetic Act. June 25, 1938, ch. 675, §1, 52 Stat. 1040.

Feuerstein, Adam. "Shift in Drug Approval Process at FDA Under Trump? Here & Now." WBUR 90.9. July 12, 2107. http://www.wbur.org/hereandnow /2017/07/12/drug-approval-process-fda-trump; accessed May 22, 2018.

Feuerstein, Adam. "Trump's FDA May be Lowering the Standards for Drug Approvals. What's the Fallout?" *STAT.* July 11, 2017. https://www .statnews.com/2017/07/11/trump-fda-gottlieb-standards/; accessed May 22, 2018.

Finkel, Adam. "Disinfecting Evidence-Based Policy Analysis of Hidden Value-Laden Constraints." *The Hastings Center Report* 48, no. 1 (2018): S21–S49.

Fiorino, D. J. "Citizen Participation and Environmental Risk: A Survey of Institutional Mechanisms." *Science, Technology & Human Values* 15, no. 2 (1990): 226–43.

Fisher, Elliott S., Julie P. Bynum, and Jonathan S. Skinner. "Slowing the Growth of Health Care Costs—Lessons from Regional Variation." *New England Journal of Medicine* 360, no. 9 (2009): 849–52.

Fleming, Thomas R. "Surrogate Endpoints and FDA's Accelerated Approval Process: The Challenges are Greater Than They Seem." *Health Affairs* 24, no. 1 (2005): 67–78.

Flexner, Abraham. "Medical Education in the United States and Canada. A Report to the Carnegie Foundation for the Advancement of Teaching." 1910. http://archive.carnegiefoundation.org/pdfs/elibrary/Carnegie_Flexner _Report.pdf; accessed May 22, 2018.

Fogel, Robert W. "The Extension of Life in Developed Countries and Its Implications for Social Policy in the Twenty-First Century." *Population and Development Review* 26 (2000): 291–317.

Fojo, Tito. "Precision Oncology: A Strategy We Were Not Ready to Deploy." *Seminars in Oncology* 43, no. 1 (2016): 9–12.

Food and Drug Administration. "Approval Package for Florbetapir F 18 Injection." April 6, 2012. https://www.accessdata.fda.gov/drugsatfda_docs /nda/2012/202008Orig1s000Approv.pdf; accessed May 22, 2018.

Food and Drug Administration. "Drug Approval Package. Harvoni." https://www .accessdata.fda.gov/drugsatfda_docs/nda/2014/205834Orig1s000TOC. cfm; Gilead, "U.S. Food and Drug Administration Approves Gilead's Harvoni® (Ledipasvir/Sofosbuvir), the First Once-Daily Single Tablet Regimen for the Treatment of Genotype 1 Chronic Hepatitis C." https://www.gilead .com/news/press-releases/2014/10/us-food-and-drug-administration -approves-gileads-harvoni-ledipasvirsofosbuvir-the-first-oncedaily-single -tablet-regimen-for-the-treatment-of-genotype-1-chronic-hepatitis-c; accessed June 9, 2018.

Food and Drug Administration. "FDA Acts to Remove Unproven, Potentially Harmful Treatment Used in 'Stem Cell' Centers Targeting Vulnerable Patients." FDA News Release. August 28, 2017. https://www.fda.gov /NewsEvents/Newsroom/PressAnnouncements/ucm573427.htm; accessed May 22, 2018.

Food and Drug Administration. "FDA Announces Comprehensive Regenerative Medicine Policy Framework." News Release. November 15, 2017. https:// www.fda.gov/NewsEvents/Newsroom/PressAnnouncements/ucm 585345.htm; accessed May 22, 2018.

Food and Drug Administration. "FDA Approves Sovaldi for Chronic Hepatitis C." FDA News Release. December 9, 2013. https://www.hhs.gov /hepatitis/blog/2013/12/09/fda-approves-sovaldi-for-chronic-hepatitis -c.html; accessed May 22, 2018.

Food and Drug Administration. "Final Agenda, Part 15 Hearing." September 12–13, 2016. https://www.fda.gov/biologicsbloodvaccines/newsevents

/workshopsmeetingsconferences/ucm509279.htm; Transcript, Part 15 Hearing. "Draft Guidances Relating to the Regulation of Human Cells, Tissues or Cellular Products." September 12, 2016. https://www.fda.gov/downloads/BiologicsBloodVaccines/NewsEvents/WorkshopsMeetingsConferences/UCM532350.pdf; September 13, 2016. https://www.fda.gov/downloads/BiologicsBloodVaccines/NewsEvents/WorkshopsMeetingsConferences/UCM532633.pdf; accessed May 22, 2018.

Food and Drug Administration. "Hearing on Proposal to Withdraw Approval for the Breast Cancer Indication for Bevacizumab (Avastin)." U.S. Department of Health and Human Services. July 6, 2011. https://www.fda.gov/NewsEvents/MeetingsConferencesWorkshops/ucm255874.htm; accessed May 22, 2018.

Food and Drug Administration. "Human Cells Tissues, and Cellular and Tissue-Based Products." *Federal Register* 55, no. 5447 (January 19, 2001): 5458 (codified at 21 CFR 1271).

Food and Drug Administration. "Human Cells, Tissues, and Cellular and Tissue-Based Products (HCT/Ps) from Adipose Tissue: Regulatory Considerations." Draft Guidance for Industry. December 2014.

Food and Drug Administration. "Minimal Manipulation of Human Cells, Tissues, and Cellular and Tissue-Based Products." Draft Guidance for Industry and Food and Drug Administration Staff. December 2014, 8.

Food and Drug Administration. [Docket No. FDA–2010–N–0621]. "Proposal to Withdraw Approval for the Breast Cancer Indication for Bevacizumab; Hearing." *Federal Register* 86, no. 91. (May 11, 2011): 27332–35. https://www.gpo.gov/fdsys/pkg/FR-2011-05-11/pdf/2011-11539.pdf#page=1; accessed May 22, 2018.

Food and Drug Administration. "Public Workshop. Scientific Evidence in Development of HCT/Ps Subject to Premarket Approval." September 8, 2016. https://www.fda.gov/downloads/BiologicsBloodVaccines/NewsEvents/WorkshopsMeetingsConferences/UCM530238.pdf; accessed May 22, 2018.

Food and Drug Administration. "Regulatory Considerations for Human Cells, Tissues, and Cellular and Tissue-Based Products: Minimal Manipulation and Homologous Use." Guidance for Industry and Food and Drug Administration Staff. November 2017 (Corrected December 2017). https://www.fda.gov/downloads/BiologicsBloodVaccines/GuidanceComplianceRegulatoryInformation/Guidances/CellularandGeneTherapy/UCM585403.pdf; accessed May 22, 2018.

Food and Drug Administration. "Same Surgical Procedure Exception under 21 CFR 1271.15(b): Questions and Answers Regarding the Scope of the Exception." Draft Guidance, October 2014.

Food and Drug Administration. "Statement from FDA Commissioner Scott Gottlieb, MD on the FDA's New Policy Steps and Enforcement Efforts to Ensure Proper Oversight of Stem Cell Therapies and Regenerative

Medicine." August 28, 2017. https://www.fda.gov/NewsEvents/Newsroom
/PressAnnouncements/ucm573443.htm; accessed May 22, 2018.

Food and Drug Administration. "Warning Letter. U.S. Stem Cell Clinic, LLC
8/24/17." August 2017. https://www.fda.gov/ICECI/EnforcementActions
/WarningLetters/2017/ucm573187.htm; accessed May 22, 2018.

Food and Drug Administration History. September 29, 2017. https://www.fda
.gov/AboutFDA/WhatWeDo/History/; accessed May 22, 2018.

Food and Drug Administration Safety and Innovation Act of 2012. Public Law
112–144.

Foote, Susan Bartlett. "Focus on Locus: Evolution of Medicare's Local Coverage
Policy." *Health Affairs* 22, no. 4 (2003): 137–46.

Foote, Susan Bartlett. "Why Medicare Cannot Promulgate a National Coverage
Rule: A Case of Regula Mortis." *Journal of Health Politics, Policy and Law* 27,
no. 5 (2002): 707–30.

Foote, Susan Bartlett, Douglas Wholey, Todd Rockwood, and Rachel Halpern.
"Resolving the Tug-of-War Between Medicare's National and Local Coverage." *Health Affairs* 23, no. 4 (2004): 108–23.

Friedman, Courtney. "Gov. Abbott Signs HB 810, Allowing Texans to Use Own
Stem Cells as Medicine." KSAT. June 13, 2017. https://www.ksat.com
/news/politics/gov-abbott-signs-hb-810-allowing-texans-to-use-own
-stem-cells-as-medicine; accessed May 22, 2018.

Fryback, D. G. and J. R. Thornbury. "The Efficacy of Diagnostic Imaging." *Medical Decision Making* 11, no. 2 (1991): 88–94.

Ghinea, Narcyz, Wendy Lipworth, Ian Kerridge, Miles Little, and Richard
O. Day. "Ethics & Evidence in Medical Debates: The Case of Recombinant Activated Factor VII." *Hastings Center Report* 44, no. 2 (2014): 38–45.

Gieryn, T. F. *Cultural Boundaries of Science: Credibility on the Line.* Chicago: University of Chicago Press, 1999.

Gillick, Muriel R. "Medicare Coverage for Technological Innovations—Time for
New Criteria?" *New England Journal of Medicine* 350, no. 21 (2004):
2199–201.

Gillick, Muriel R. "The Technological Imperative and the Battle for the Hearts of
America." *Perspectives in Biology and Medicine* 50, no. 2 (2007): 276–94.

Ginsberg, Seth D. "What to Do if You're Denied Coverage for a New Cholesterol
Drug You Need." *U.S. News & World Report.* September 9, 2016. http://
health.usnews.com/health-news/patient-advice/articles/2016-09-09
/what-to-do-if-youre-denied-coverage-for-a-new-cholesterol-drug-you
-need; accessed May 22, 2018.

Gold, Richard H., Lawrence W. Bassett, and Bobbi Widoff. "Highlights from the
History of Mammography." *Radiographics* 10 (1990): 1111–31.

Goldman, Lea. "The Big Business of Breast Cancer." *Marie Claire.* September 14,
2011. http://www.marieclaire.com/politics/news/a6506/breast-cancer
-business-scams/; accessed May 22, 2018.

Gotink, K. J. and H. M. Verheul. "Anti-Angiogenic Tyrosine Kinase Inhibitors:
What Is Their Mechanism of Action?" *Angiogenesis* 13, no. 1 (2010): 1–14.

Gottlieb, Scott. "Examining Patient Access to Investigational Drugs." Testimony before the Subcommittee on Health, Committee on Energy and Commerce, U.S. House of Representatives. October 3, 2017. https://www.fda.gov/NewsEvents/Testimony/ucm578634.htm; accessed May 22, 2018.

Gottlieb, Scott and Coleen Klasmeier. "The FDA Wants to Regulate Your Cells." AEI.org. August 8, 2012. http://www.aei.org/article/health/the-fda-wants-to-regulate-your-cells/; accessed May 22, 2018.

Government Accountability Office. "DRUG SAFETY: FDA Expedites Many Applications, but Data for Postapproval Oversight Need Improvement." Report to the Ranking Member, Subcommittee on Labor, Health and Human Services, Education, and Related Agencies, Committee on Appropriations, House of Representatives, GAO-16-1. Washington, D.C.: Government Accountability Office, December 2015.

Government Accountability Office. "Medical Device Companies: Trends in Reported Net Sales and Profits Before and After Implementation of the Patient Protection and Affordable Care Act," (GAO-15-635R: Published: June 30, 2015. Publicly Released: July 30, 2015. https://www.gao.gov/products/GAO-15-635R; accessed May 22, 2018.

Graf, M. D., D. F. Needham, N. Teed, and T. Brown. "Genetic Testing Insurance Coverage Trends: A Review of Publicly Available Policies from the Largest U.S. Payers." *Personalized Medicine* 10, no. 3 (2013): 235–43.

Gray, Bradford H. "The Legislative Battle Over Health Services Research." *Health Affairs* 11, no. 4 (1992): 38–66.

Gray, Bradford H., Michael K. Gusmano, and Sara R. Collins. "AHCPR and the Politics of Health Services Research." *Health Affairs Web Exclusive* (2003): W3283–W307.

Grayson, Charlotte. "New Approaches to Chemotherapy for Breast Cancer." *MedicineNet.com*. September 7, 2002. http://www.medicinenet.com/script/main/art.asp?articlekey=51886; accessed May 22, 2018.

Greenhalgh, Trisha, Jeremy Howick, and Neal Naskrey, for the Evidence-Based Medicine Renaissance Group. "Evidence-Based Medicine: A Movement in Crisis?" *BMJ* 348 (2014): g3725.

Griffith, Morgan. "Congressman Griffith's Weekly E-Newsletter 5.5.14." https://morgangriffith.house.gov/news/documentsingle.aspx?DocumentID=378942; accessed May 22, 2018.

Grob, Rachel. *Testing Baby: The Transformation of Newborn Screening, Parenting, and Policymaking.* New Brunswick, NJ: Rutgers University Press, 2011.

Gusmano, Michael K. "FDA Decisions and Public Deliberation: Challenges and Opportunities." *Public Administration Review* 73, no. S1 (2013): S115–S126.

Gusmano, Michael K. "Health Systems Performance and the Politics of Cancer Survival." *World Medical & Health Policy* 5, no. 1 (2013): 76–84.

Gusmano, Michael K. and Daniel Callahan. "Value for Money: Use with Care." *Annals of Internal Medicine* 154, no. 3 (2011): 207–08.

Gusmano, Michael K. and Gregory E. Kaebnick. "Clarifying the Role of Values in Cost-Effectiveness." *Health Economics, Policy and Law* 11, no. 4 (2016): 439–43.

Gusmano, Michael K., Victor G. Rodwin, and Daniel Weisz. "Persistent Inequalities in Health and Access to Health Services: Evidence from NYC." *World Medical & Health Policy* 9, no. 2 (2017): 186–205.

Gusmano, Michael K. and Mark Schlesinger. "The Social Roles of Medicare: Assessing Medicare's Collateral Benefits." *Journal of Health, Politics, Policy and Law* 26, no. 1 (2001): 37–81.

Gusmano, Michael K., Mark Schlesinger, and Tracey Thomas. "Policy Feedback and Public Opinion: The Role of Employer Responsibility in Social Policy." *Journal of Health Politics, Policy, and Law* 27, no. 5 (2002): 731–72.

Gusmano, Michael K., Marc Suhrcke, Ellen Nolte, Martin McKee, Victor G. Rodwin, and Daniel Weisz. "Health Care as an Investment? Reframing the Health Policy Debates in Europe." *Alliance for Health & the Future.* Issue Brief 3, no. 1 (2008): 1–7.

Guthman, Julie and Sandy Brown. "Whose Life Counts Biopolitics and the 'Bright Line' of Chloropicrin Mitigation in California's Strawberry Industry." *Science, Technology & Human Values* 41, no. 3 (2015): 1–22.

Guyatt, Gordon, Elie A. Akl, Jack Hirsh, Clive Kearon, Mark Crowther, David Gutterman, Sandra Zelman Lewis, Ian Nathanson, Roman Jaeschke, and Holger Schnemann. "The Vexing Problem of Guidelines and Conflict of Interest: A Potential Solution." *Annals of Internal Medicine* 152, no. 11 (2010): 738–41.

Hadler, Nortin. "Does Screening Mammography Save Lives?" *ABC News.* May 21, 2007. http://abcnews.go.com/Health/OnCallPlus/story?id=3196417; accessed May 22, 2018.

Hall, Peter A. "Policy Paradigms: Social Learning and the State: The Case of Economic Policymaking in Britain." *Comparative Politics* 25, no. 3 (1993): 275–96.

Hall, Peter A. "The Role of Interests, Institutions and Ideas in the Comparative Political Economy of the Industrialized Nations." In *Comparative Politics: Rationality, Culture, and Structure*, edited by Mark Irving Lichbach and Alan S. Zuckerman, 174–207. New York: Cambridge University Press, 1997.

Hall, Peter A. and Rosemary C. R. Taylor. "Political Science and the Three New Institutionalisms." *Political Studies* 44, no. 5 (1996): 936–57.

Handfield, Robert and Josh Feldstein. "Insurance Companies' Perspectives on the Orphan Drug Pipeline." *American Health & Drug Benefits* 6, no. 9 (2013): 589–98.

Harris, Richard. "R&D Costs for Cancer Drugs Are Likely Much Less Than Industry Claims, Study Finds." *NPR, WNYC Radio.* September 11, 2017. https://www.npr.org/sections/health-shots/2017/09/11/550135932/r-d-costs-for-cancer-drugs-are-likely-much-less-than-industry-claims-study-finds; accessed May 22, 2018.

HCFA. "Medicare Program, Criteria for Making Coverage Decisions." *Federal Register* 65, no. 95 (200): 31124–29, at 31127.

Healy, Bernadine. "FNS." November 23, 2009, transcript. http://www.foxnews .com/story/2009/11/23/transcript-dr-bernadine-healy-on-fns.html; accessed May 22, 2018.

Heather, Douglas. "Politics and Science: Untangling Values, Ideologies, and Reasons." *Annals of the American Academy of Political and Social Science* 658 (2015): 296–306.

Heclo, Hugh. *Modern Social Politics in Britain and Sweden: From Relief to Income Maintenance.* New Haven, CT: Yale University Press, 1987.

HemOne Today. "USPSTF Breast Cancer Screening Recommendations Remain Unchanged Despite Controversy." *HemOne Today.* January 11, 2016. https://www.healio.com/hematology-oncology/breast-cancer/news/in -the-journals/%7B4e79de36-911d-41ef-bed3-3ad171be2f26%7D/uspstf -breast-cancer-screening-recommendations-remain-unchanged-despite -controversy; accessed May 22, 2018.

Hep Magazine. "Missouri Is the Latest State to Roll Back Restrictions on Hepatitis C Treatment." December 1, 2017. https://www.hepmag.com/article /missouri-latest-state-roll-back-restrictions-hepatitis-c-treatment; accessed May 22, 2018.

Herper, M. "The FDA's Cancer Czar Says He Can't Approve New Drugs Fast Enough." *Forbes.* June 23, 2013. www.forbes.com/sites/matthewherper /2013/06/23/the-fdas-cancer-czarsays-he-cant-approve-new-drugs-fast -enough/; accessed May 22, 2018.

Herszenhorn, David M. "Senate Blocks the Use of New Mammography Guidelines." *New York Times.* December 3, 2009. https://prescriptions.blogs .nytimes.com/2009/12/03/gop-amendments-aim-at-new-cancer -guidelines/; accessed May 22, 2018.

Hillman, Bruce J. *A Plague on All Our Houses: Medical Intrigue, Hollywood, and the Discovery of AIDS.* Lebanon, NH: ForeEdge, 2016.

Hillman, Bruce J., Richard A. Frank, and Brian C. Abraham. "The Medical Imaging & Technology Alliance Conference on Research Endpoints Appropriate for Medicare Coverage of New PET Radiopharmaceuticals." *Journal of Nuclear Medicine* 54, no. 9 (2013): 1675–1679.

Hillman, Bruce J., Richard A. Frank, and Gail M. Rodriguez. "New Pathways to Medicare Coverage for Innovative PET Radiopharmaceuticals: Report of a Medical Imaging & Technology Alliance (MITA) Workshop." *Journal of Nuclear Medicine* 53, no. 2 (2012): 336–42.

Hirschman, J., S. Whitman, and D. Ansell. "The Black: White Disparity in Breast Cancer Mortality: The Example of Chicago." *Cancer Causes & Control* 18, no. 3 (2007): 323–33.

Hoffer et al. v. Jones. Case 4:17-cv-00214-MW-CAS Document 185, U.S. District Court for the Northern District of Florida. Filed December 13, 2017.

Hoover Institution. "TAKE IT TO THE LIMITS: Milton Friedman on Libertarianism." *Uncommon Knowledge.* 2010. https://www.hoover.org

/research/take-it-limits-milton-friedman-libertarianism; accessed May 22, 2018.

Hopkins, Virginia. "Mammogram Controversy—Follow the Money." *Health Watchers' News and Views.* November 18, 2009. http://www.healthwatchersnews.com/2009/11/mammogram-controversy-follow-the-money/; accessed May 22, 2018.

Howard, D. H. "Quality and Consumer Choice in Healthcare: Evidence from Kidney Transplantation." *Topics in Economic Analysis and Policy* 5, no. 1 (2005): 1–20.

Howard, Paul. "To Lower Drug Prices, Innovate, Don't Regulate." *New York Times.* September 23, 2015. https://www.nytimes.com/roomfordebate/2015/09 /23/should-the-government-impose-drug-price-controls/to-lower-drug -prices-innovate-dont-regulate; accessed May 22, 2018.

Hresko, A. and S. B. Haga. "Insurance Coverage Policies for Personalized Medicine." *Journal of Personalized Medicine* 2, no. 4 (2012): 201–16. PMCID: PMC4251376.

Hunt, Bijou R., Steve Whitman, and Marc S. Hurlbert. "Increasing Black:White Disparities in Breast Cancer Mortality in the 50 Largest Cities in the United States." *Cancer Epidemiology* 38, no. 2 (2014): 118–23.

Hyun, Insoo. "Allowing Innovative Stem Cell-Based Therapies Outside of Clinical Trials: Ethical and Policy Challenges." *Journal of Law, Medicine & Ethics* 38, no. 2 (2010): 277–85.

IDEAS. "Imaging Dementia—Evidence for Amyloid Scanning." https://www .ideas-study.org/about/history/; accessed May 22, 2018.

IDEAS. "Interim Results from the IDEAS Study Reported at AAIC 2017 in London." https://www.ideas-study.org/2017/07/20/interim-results-from-the -ideas-study-reported-at-aaic-2017-in-london/; accessed May 22, 2018.

IDEAS. "Protocol." https://www.ideas-study.org/referring-physicians/protocol/; accessed May 22, 2018.

Iglehart, John K. "The Political Fight Over Comparative Effectiveness Research." *Health Affairs* 29, no. 10 (2010): 1757–60.

Iglehart, John K. "Prioritizing Comparative-Effectiveness Research—IOM Recommendations." *New England Journal of Medicine* 361, no. 4 (2009): 325–28.

Illich, Ivan. *Medical Nemesis: The Expropriation of Health.* London: Calder & Boyars, 1974.

Immergut, Ellen M. *Health Politics: Interests and Institutions in Western Europe.* Cambridge: CUP Archive, 1992.

Institute of Medicine. *Crossing the Quality Chasm: New Health System for the 21st Century.* Washington, D.C.: National Academies Press, 2001.

Institute of Medicine. *Evidence-Based Medicine and the Changing Nature of Healthcare: Meeting Summary.* Washington, D.C.: National Academies Press, 2008.

Institute of Medicine. *Initial National Priorities for Comparative Effectiveness Research.* Washington, D.C.: National Academies Press, 2009.

Institute of Medicine. *Medicare: A Strategy for Quality Assurance, Volume I.* Washington, D.C.: National Academies Press, 1990.

Institute of Medicine. *To Err is Human: Building a Safer Health System.* Washington, D.C.: National Academies Press, 1999.

International Society for Stem Cell Research. "ISSCR Opposes REGROW Act." September 15, 2016. http://www.isscr.org/professional-resources/news -publicationsss/isscr-news-articles/article-listing/2016/09/15/isscr -opposes-the-regrow-act; accessed May 22, 2018.

Jack, Clifford R., Marilyn S. Albert, David S. Knopman, Guy M. McKhann, Reisa A. Sperling, Maria C. Carrillo, Bill Thies, and Creighton H. Phelps. "Introduction to the Recommendations from the National Institute on Aging-Alzheimer's Association Workgroups on Diagnostic Guidelines for Alzheimer's Disease." *Alzheimer's & Dementia* 7, no. 3 (2011): 257–62.

Jagpreet, Chatwal, Fasiha Kanwal, Mark S. Roberts, and Michael A. Dunn. "Cost-Effectiveness and Budget Impact of Hepatitis C Virus Treatment with Sofosbuvir and Ledipasvir in the United States." *Annals of Internal Medicine* 162, no. 6 (2015): 397–406. doi:10.7326/M14-1336.

Jatoi, Ismail and Anthony B. Miller. "Why Is Breast Cancer Mortality Declining?" *The Lancet Oncology* 4, no. 4 (2003): 251–54.

Jewell, Christopher and Lisa Bero. "Public Participation and Claimsmaking: Evidence Utilization and Divergent Policy Frames in California's Ergonomics Rulemaking." *Journal of Public Administration Research and Theory* 17, no. 4 (2007): 625–50.

Jogerst, M. A. *Reform in the House of Commons: The Select Committee System.* Lexington, NY: University of Kentucky Press, 1993.

Johnson, Carolyn Y. and Brady Dennis. "How an $84,000 Drug Got Its Price: 'Let's Hold Our Position . . . Whatever the Headlines.'" *Washington Post.* December 1, 2015. https://www.washingtonpost.com/news/wonk/wp/2015/12/01 /how-an-84000-drug-got-its-price-lets-hold-our-position-whatever-the -headlines/?utm_term=.cc34a100501d; accessed May 22, 2018.

Johnson, Keith A., Satoshi Minoshima, Nicolaas I. Bohnen, Kevin J. Donohoe, Norman L. Foster, Peter Herscovitch, Jason H. Karlawish, Christopher C. Rowe, Maria C. Carrillo, Dean M. Hartley, Saima Hedrick, Virginia Pappas, and William H. Thies. "Appropriate Use Criteria for Amyloid PET: A Report of the Amyloid Imaging Task Force, the Society of Nuclear Medicine and Molecular Imaging, and the Alzheimer's Association." *Journal of Nuclear Medicine* 54, no. 3 (2013): 476–90.

Johnson, Keith A., Satoshi Minoshima, Nicolaas I. Bohnen, Kevin J. Donohoe, Norman L. Foster, Peter Herscovitch, Jason H. Karlawish, Christopher C. Rowe, Saima Hedrick, Virginia Pappas, Maria C. Carrillo, and Dean Hartley. "Update on Appropriate Use Criteria for Amyloid PET Imaging: Dementia Experts, Mild Cognitive Impairment, and Education." *Journal of Nuclear Medicine* 54, no. 7 (2013): 1011–13.

Joseph, Andrew. "After Criticism from Scientists, Congress Eases Its Pursuit of Faster Stem Cell Therapies." *STAT.* November 20, 2016. https://www.statnews.com/2016/11/30/stem-cells-cures-act/; accessed May 22, 2018.

Juran, J. M. *A History of Managing for Quality.* Milwaukee, WI: ASQC Quality Press, 1995.

Kaebnick, Gregory E. and Michael K. Gusmano. "CBA and Precaution: Policy-Making about Emerging Technologies." *Hastings Center Report* 48, no. 1 (2018): S88–S96.

Kahneman, Daniel and Amos Tversky. "Advances in Prospect Theory: Cumulative Representation of Uncertainty." *Journal of Risk and Uncertainty* 5, no. 4 (1992): 297–323.

Kalager, Mette, Magnus Løberg, Vinjar M. Fønnebø, and Michael Bretthauer. "Failure to Account for Selection-Bias." *International Journal of Cancer* 113, no. 11 (2013): 2751–53.

Kanavos, Panos, Allessandra Ferrario, Sotiris Vandoros, and Gerard F. Anderson. "Higher U.S. Branded Drug Prices and Spending Compared to Other Countries May Stem Partly from Quick Uptake of New Drugs." *Health Affairs* 32, no. 4 (2013): 753–61.

Kaplan, Sheila. "Trump Derides 'Slow and Burdensome' Approval Process at FDA." STAT. February 28, 2017. https://www.statnews.com/2017/02/28/trump-address-rare-disease-drugs/; accessed May 22, 2018.

Karlawish, Jason. "Addressing the Ethical, Policy, and Social Challenges of Preclinical Alzheimer Disease." *Neurology* 77, no. 15 (2011): 1487–93.

Karlin-Smith, Sarah. "New Stem Cell Legislation Raises Alarm." Politico. May 2, 2016. https://www.politico.com/tipsheets/prescription-pulse/2016/05/new-legislation-on-stem-cells-raises-alarm-214069; accessed May 22, 2018.

Karlin-Smith, Sarah and Seung Min Kim. "Senate Approves 'Right-to-Try' Drug Bill." August 3, 2017. Politico. https://www.politico.com/story/2017/08/03/senate-right-to-try-drug-bill-241293; accessed May 22, 2018.

Kaufman, S. R. and L. Fjord. "Medicare, Ethics, and Reflexive Longevity." *Medical Anthropology Quarterly* 25, no. 2 (2011): 209–31.

Keller, A. C. and L. Packel. "Going for the Cure: Patient Interest Groups and Health Advocacy in the United States." *Journal of Health Politics, Policy and Law* 39, no. 2 (2014): 331–67.

Kelley, Stanley. *Professional Public Relations and Political Power.* Baltimore, MD: Johns Hopkins University Press, 1956.

Kesselheim, Aaron S. "Trends in Utilization of FDA Expedited Drug Development and Approval Programs, 1987–2014: Cohort Study." *BMJ* (2015): 351. doi: https://doi.org/10.1136/bmj.h4633; accessed May 22, 2018.

Kesselheim, Aaron S., Tina Yongtian Tan, Jonathan J. Darrow, and Jerry Avorn. "Existing FDA Pathways Have Potential to Ensure Early Access to, and Appropriate Use of, Specialty Drugs." *Health Affairs* 30, no. 10 (2014): 1770–78.

Kessler, David A. "The Regulation of Investigational Drugs." *New England Journal of Medicine* 320, no. 5 (1989): 281–88, 283.

King, Samantha. *Pink Ribbons, Inc.: Breast Cancer and the Politics of Philanthropy.* Minneapolis: University of Minnesota Press, 2006.

Kleutghen, Paul, David Mitchell, Aaron S. Kesselheim, Mehdi Najafzadeh, and Ameet Sarpatwari. "Drugs Don't Work if People Can't Afford Them: The High Price of Tisagenlecleucel." Health Affairs Blog. February 8, 2018. https://www.healthaffairs.org/do/10.1377/hblog20180205.292531/full/; accessed May 22, 2018.

Knoepfler, Paul. "Neuralstem Flirting with Stem Cell Noncompliance in Colorado via Right to Try Law?" The Niche. Knoepfler Lab Stem Cell Blog. June 11, 2014. https://ipscell.com/2014/06/neuralstem-flirting-with-stem-cell-noncompliance-in-colorado-via-right-to-try-law/; accessed May 22, 2018.

Kolata, Gina. "Medicare Covering New Treatments with a Catch." *New York Times.* November 5, 2004. http://query.nytimes.com/gst/fullpage.html?res=9A02E3DF153CF936A35752C1A9629C8B63&pagewanted=all; accessed May 22, 2018.

Kort v. Burwell. U.S. District Court for the District of Columbia, Civil No. 1:14-cv-0159 (APM). Memorandum Opinion. July 19, 2016, 31.

Kramer, D. B. and A. S. Kesselheim. "Coverage of Magnetic Resonance Imaging for Patients with Cardiac Devices: Improving the Coverage with Evidence Development Program." *Journal of the American Medical Association Cardiology* 2 (2017): 711–12.

Kuriyan, Ajay E., Thomas A. Albini, Justin H. Townsend, Marianeli Rodriguez, Hemang K. Pandya, Robert E. Leonard II, M. Brandon Parrott, Philip J. Rosenfeld, Harry W. Flynn Jr., and Jeffrey L. Goldberg. "Vision Loss after Intravitreal Injection of Autologous 'Stem Cells' for AMD." *New England Journal of Medicine* 376, no. 11 (2017): 1047–53.

LaMattina, John. "Gilead's CEO Admits to 'Failures' in Setting Price of $1,000-a-Pill Breakthrough." *Forbes.* December 8, 2016. https://www.forbes.com/sites/johnlamattina/2016/12/08/gileads-ceo-apologetic-about-sovaldis-1000-per-pill-price-tag/#6d58bc431a97; accessed May 22, 2018.

Lau, Darren, Ubaka Ogbogu, Benjamin Taylor, Tania Stafinski, Devidas Menon, and Timothy Caulfield. "Stem Cell Clinics Online: The Direct-to-Consumer Portrayal of Stem Cell Medicine." *Cell Stem Cell* 3, no. 6 (2008): 591–94.

Lavertu, Stéphane, Daniel E. Walters, and David L. Weimer. "Scientific Expertise and the Balance of Political Interests: MEDCAC and Medicare Coverage Decisions." *Journal of Public Administration Research and Theory* 22, no. 1 (2011): 55–81.

Law, Marc and Gary D. Libecap. "The Determinants of Progressive Era Reform. The Pure Food and Drugs Act of 1906." In *Corruption and Reform: Lessons from America's Economic History*, edited by Edward L. Glaeser and Claudia Goldin, 319–41. Chicago: University of Chicago Press, 2006.

Lenzer, Jeanne. "Is the United States Preventive Services Task Force Still a Voice of Caution?" *BMJ* 356 (2017): j743. doi: 10.1136/bmj.j743.

Lerner, Baron. *Breast Cancer Wars: Hope, Fear and the Pursuit of a Cure in Twenty-First Century America*. Oxford: Oxford University Press, 2001.

Lidbrink, E., J. Elfving, and E. Jonsonn. "Neglected Aspects of False Positive Findings of Mammography in Breast Cancer Screening: Analysis of False Positive Cases from the Stockholm Trial." *BMJ* 312 (1996): 273–76.

Light, Donald W. and Joel Lexchin. "Why Do Cancer Drugs Get Such an Easy Ride?" *BMJ* 350 (2015): h2068. doi:10.1136/bmj.h2068.

Lillvis, Denise F., Anna Kirkland, and Anna Frick. "Power and Persuasion in the Vaccine Debates: An Analysis of Political Efforts and Outcomes in the United States, 1998–2012." *Milbank Quarterly* 92, no.3 (2014): 475–508.

Lilly. "Lilly Disappointed in Medicare Decision to Deny Appropriate Patient Access to Beta-Amyloid Imaging Agents, Including Amyvid™ (Florbetapir F 18 Injection), Despite Support From Experts, Patients, and the Alzheimer's Disease Community." September 27, 2013. https://investor.lilly.com/releasedetail.cfm?releaseid=793700; accessed May 22, 2018.

Lilly USA, LLC. "Request for Reconsideration of Medical National Coverage Determinations Manual." § 220.6, "Positron Emission Tomography (PET) Scans." 2012. https://www.cms.gov/Medicare/Coverage/Determination-Process/downloads/id265.pdf; accessed May 22, 2018.

Lindblom, Charles E. *Politics and Markets*. New York: Basic Books, 1977.

Lindvall, Olle and Insoo Hyun. "Medical Innovation versus Stem Cell Tourism." *Science* 324, no. 5935 (2009): 1664–65.

Litman, Theodor J. and Leonard S. Robins. *Health Politics and Policy*, 2nd edition. New York: Delmar Series in Health Services Administration, 1991.

Lo Re III, Vincent, Charitha Gowda, Paul N. Urick, Joshua T. Halladay, Amanda Binkley, Dena M. Carbonari, Kathryn Battista, Cassandra Peleckis, Jody Gilmore, Jason A. Roy, Jalpa A. Doshi, Peter P. Reese, Rajender Reddy, and Jay R. Kostman. "Disparities in Absolute Denial of Modern Hepatitis C Therapy by Type of Insurance." *Clinical Gastroenterology and Hepatology* 14, no. 7 (2016): 1035–43.

Luce, Bryan and Rebecca Singer Cohen. "Health Technology Assessment in the United States." *International Journal of Technology Assessment in Health Care* 25, Suppl. 1 (2009): 33–41.

Maienschein, Jane. "Regenerative Medicine's Historical Roots in Regeneration, Transplantation, and Translation." *Developmental Biology* 358, no. 2 (2011): 278–84.

Makary, Martin A. and Michael Daniel. "Medical Error—The Third Leading Cause of Death in the US." *BMJ* 353 (2016): i2139. doi: 10.1136/bmj.i2139.

Maloney, S. "AHRQ Prevention Program—Opportunity for Public Comment." April 16, 2010. updates@subscriptions.ahrq.gov; accessed May 22, 2018.

Manns, M. P., H. Wedemeyer, and M. Cornber. "Treating Viral Hepatitis C: Efficacy, Side Effects, and Complications." *Gut* 55 (2006): 1350–59.

Marks, Harry M. *The Progress of Experiment: Science and Therapeutic Reform in the United States, 1900–1990.* Cambridge: Cambridge University Press, 2000.

Marmor, Theodore. *The Politics of Medicare.* Chicago: Aldine Publishing Company, 1973.

Marmor, Theodore, Richard Freeman, and Kieke Okma. "Comparative Perspectives and Policy Learning in the World of Health Care." *Journal of Comparative Policy* 7, no. 4 (2005): 331–48.

Marmor, Theodore, Jonathan Oberlander, and Joseph White. "The Obama Administration's Options for Health Care Cost Control: Hope Versus Reality." *Annals of Internal Medicine* 150, no. 7 (2009): 485–89.

Maschke, Karen J. and Michael K. Gusmano. "Evidence and Access to Biomedical Interventions: The Case of Stem Cell Treatments." *Journal of Health Politics, Policy and Law* 41, no. 5 (2016): 917–36.

Maschke, Karen J., Michael K. Gusmano, and Mildred Z. Solomon. "Expensive Breakthrough Treatments: The Case of CAR-T Cell Cancer Treatment." *Health Affairs* 36, no. 10 (2017): 1698–1700.

McCaughan, Michael. "Health Policy Brief: Expedited Approval Pathways." *Health Affairs.* July 21, 2017. doi: 10.1377/hpb2017.2.

McCright Aaron M, Katherine Dentzman, Meghan Charters, and Thomas Dietz. "The Influence of Political Ideology on Trust in Science." *Environmental Research Letters* 8, no. 4 (2013): 044029.

McGinley, Laurie. "FDA Cracks Down on Stem-Cell Clinics, Including One Using Smallpox Vaccine in Cancer Patients." *Washington Post.* August 28, 2017. https://www.washingtonpost.com/news/to-your-health/wp/2017/08/28/fda-cracks-down-on-stem-cell-clinics-including-one-using-smallpox-vaccine-in-cancer-patients/?utm_term=.67b4aa33d45d&wpisrc=al_alert-hse&wpmk=1; accessed May 22, 2018.

McGinley, Laurie and Carolyn Y. Johnson. "Trump to Select Scott Gottlieb, a Physician with Deep Drug Industry Ties, To Run the FDA." *Washington Post.* March 10, 2017. https://www.washingtonpost.com/news/to-your-health/wp/2017/03/10/trump-selects-scott-gottlieb-a-physician-with-deep-drug-industry-ties-to-run-the-fda/?utm_term=.72e452e90b75; accessed May 22, 2018.

McKhann, Guy M., David S. Knopman, Howard Chertkow, Bradley T. Hyman, Clifford R. Jack Jr., Claudia H. Kawas, William E. Klunk, Walter J. Koroshetz, Jennifer J. Manly, Richard Mayeux, Richard C. Mohs, John C. Morris, Martin N. Rossor, Philip Scheltens, Maria C. Carrillo, Bill Thies, Sandra Weintraub, and Creighton H. Phelps. "The Diagnosis of Dementia Due to Alzheimer's Disease: Recommendations from the National Institute on Aging-Alzheimer's Association Workgroups on Diagnostic Guidelines for Alzheimer's Disease." *Alzheimer's & Dementia* 7, no. 3 (2011): 263–69.

Medical Device Innovation Consortium. "Medical Device Innovation Consortium (MDIC) Patient Centered Benefit-Risk Project Report." n.d. http://mdic.org/wp-content/uploads/2015/05/MDIC_Summary_Report_SinglePage_5.7.15.pdf; accessed May 22, 2018.

Meltzer, David and James Magnus. "Inconsistencies in the 'Societal Perspective' on Costs of the Panel on Cost-Effectiveness in Health and Medicine." *Medical Decision Making*, 19, no. 4 (1999): 371–77.

Menon, D. and T. Stafinski. "Engaging the Public in Priority-Setting for Health Technology Assessment: Findings from a Citizens' Jury." *Health Expectations* 11 (2088): 282–93.

Mershon, Erin. "Pence Says that Congress Should Get Right-to-Try Legislation 'DONE.'" STAT. January 18, 2018. https://www.statnews.com/2018/01/18/mike-pence-right-to-try/; accessed May 22, 2018.

Michael J. Fox Foundation for Parkinson's Disease. "MJFF Signs Letter Opposing the REGROW Act." Foxfeed Blog. May 21, 2016. https://www.michaeljfox.org/foundation/news-detail.php?mjff-signs-letter-opposing-the-regrow-act; accessed May 22, 2018.

Michiels, S., E. D. Saad, and M. Buyse. "Progression-Free Survival as a Surrogate for Overall Survival in Clinical Trials of Targeted Therapy in Advanced Solid Tumors." *Drugs* 77, no. 7 (2017): 713–19.

Mol, B. W., J. G. Lijmer, J. L. Evers, and P. M. Bossuyt. "Characteristics of Good Diagnostic Tests." *Seminars in Reproductive Medicine* 21, no. 1, (2003): 17–25.

Molchan, S. "A Tale of Two Conferences." *Journal of the American Medical Association Internal Medicine* 174, no. 6 (2014): 856–57.

Moon, Marilyn. *Medicare Now and in the Future.* Washington, D.C.: The Urban Institute Press, 1993.

Moons, Michelle. "Mike Pence: 'We Need Every Republican in Congress,' Every American for Healthcare 'Battle.'" *Breitbart News.* March 11, 2017. http://www.breitbart.com/big-government/2017/03/11/pence-need-every-republican-congress-every-american-healthcare-battle/; accessed May 22, 2018.

Morone, James. *The Democratic Wish: Popular Participation and the Limits of American Democracy.* New York: Basic Books, 1990.

Mundy, Alicia. "New Breast Screening Limits Face Reversal." *The Wall Street Journal.* January 12, 2010. https://www.wsj.com/articles/SB126325763413725559; accessed May 22, 2018.

Muntasell, Aura, Mariona Cabo, Sonia Servitja, Ignasi Tusquets, María Martínez-García, Ana Roviral, Federico Rojo, Joan Albanell, Miguel López-Botet1. "Interplay between Natural Killer Cells and Anti-HER2 Antibodies: Perspectives for Breast Cancer Immunotherapy." *Frontiers in Immunology* 8 (2017): 1544. doi: 10.3389/fimmu.2017.01544.

Myers, Evan R., Patricia Moorman, Jennifer M. Gierisch, Laura J. Havrilesky, Lars J. Grimm, Sujata Ghate, Brittany Davidson, Ranee Chatterjee

Mongtomery, Matthew J. Crowley, Douglas C. McCrory, Amy Kendrick, and Gillian D. Sanders. "Benefits and Harms of Breast Cancer Screening: A Systematic Review." *Journal of the American Medical Association* 314, no. 15 (2015): 1615–34.

National Cancer Institute. "High-Dose Chemotherapy." http://www.cancer.gov/cancertopics/high-dose-chemo; accessed May 22, 2018.

National Cancer Institute. "Surveillance, Epidemiology, and End Results Program." https://seer.cancer.gov/; accessed June 9, 2018.

National Geographic. "The War on Science." February 17, 2015. http://ngm.nationalgeographic.com/2015/03/science-doubters/achenbach-text; accessed May 22, 2018.

National Institutes of Health. "Stem Cell Basics." https://stemcells.nih.gov/info/basics.htm; accessed May 22, 2018.

National Institutes of Health Consensus Development Panel. "National Institutes of Health Consensus Development Conference Statement: Breast Cancer Screening for Women Ages 40–49, January 21–23, 1997." *JNCI: Journal of the National Cancer Institute* 89, no. 14 (1997): 960–65.

National Pharmaceutical Council. "Health Affairs CER Briefing Highlights Key Issues." National Pharmaceutical Council Newsletter. October 2010. http://www.npcnow.org/newsroom/commentary/health-affairs-cer-briefing-highlights-key-issues; accessed May 22, 2018.

National Research Council. *Public Engagement on Genetically Modified Organisms: When Science and Citizens Connect: Workshop Summary.* Washington, D.C.: National Academies Press, 2015.

National Research Council and Institute of Medicine. *Stem Cells and the Future Regenerative Medicine.* Washington, D.C.: National Academy Press, 2002.

Neumann, Peter J., A. B. Rosen, and M. C. Weinstein. "Medicare and Cost-Effectiveness Analysis." *New England Journal of Medicine* 353, no. 14 (2005): 1516–22.

Neumann, Peter J. and Sean R. Tunis. "Medicare and Medical Technology—The Growing Demand for Relevant Outcomes." *New England Journal of Medicine* 362, no. 5 (2010): 377–79.

New England Healthcare Institute. *Balancing Act: Comparative Effectiveness Research and Innovation in U.S. Health Care*—A White Paper. April 2009, 2.

Nisbet, Eric C., Kathryn E. Cooper, and Garrett R. Kelly. "The Partisan Brain: How Dissonant Science Messages Lead Conservatives and Liberals to (Dis)trust Science." *The Annals of the American Academy of Political and Social Science* 658, no. 1 (2015): 36–66.

Nisbet, Matthew and Ezra M. Markowitz. "Understanding Public Opinion in Debates Over Biomedical Research: Looking Beyond Political Partisanship to Focus on Beliefs about Science and Society." *PLoS One* 9, no. 2 (2014): e88473.

Oberlander, Jonathan. *The Political Life of Medicare.* Chicago: University of Chicago Press, 2003.

OECD. "OECD Health Statistics 2014: How Does the United States Compare?" http://www.oecd.org/unitedstates/Briefing-Note-UNITED -STATES-2014.pdf; accessed May 22, 2018.

Office of Inspector General, U.S. Department of Health and Human Services. "Local Coverage Determinations Create Inconsistency in Medicare Coverage." January 2014. http://oig.hhs.gov/oei/reports/oei-01-11-00500.pdf; accessed May 22, 2018.

O'Kane, Margaret. "Increasing Transparency on Health Care Costs, Coverage, and Quality." Testimony before the Senate Commerce, Science & Transportation Committee. February 27, 2013.

Ollove, Michael. "Are States Obligated to Provide Expensive Hepatitis C Drugs?" *The PEW Charitable Trusts.* February 9, 2016. http://www.pewtrusts.org /en/research-and-analysis/blogs/stateline/2016/02/09/are -states-obligated-to-provide-expensive-hepatitis-c-drugs; accessed May 22, 2018.

Otero, Hansel Javier, James D. Chambers, Brian W. Bresnahan, Maki S. Kamae, Kent E. Yuce, and Peter J. Neumann. "Medicare's National Coverage Determinations in Diagnostic Radiology: Examining Evidence and Setting Limits." *Academic Radiology* 19, no. 9 (2012): 1060–65.

Our Bodies, Ourselves. https://www.ourbodiesourselves.org/publications/our -bodies-ourselves-2011/introduction/; accessed May 22, 2018.

Pace, Lydia E. and Nancy L. Keating. "A Systematic Assessment of Benefits and Risks to Guide Breast Cancer Screening Decisions." *Journal of the American Medical Association* 311, no. 13 (2014): 1327–35.

Partridge, Anne H. and Eric P. Winer. "On Mammography—More Agreement Than Disagreement." *New England Journal of Medicine* 361, no. 26 (2009): 2499–2501.

Patashnik, Eric. "Here Are the 5 Reasons Republicans Are Trying to Cut Research on Evidence-Based Medicine." *Washington Post.* October 22, 2015. https:// www.washingtonpost.com/news/monkey-cage/wp/2015/06/22/here -are-the-5-reasons-republicans-are-trying-to-cut-research-on-evidence -based-medicine/?utm_term=.c0543444b649; accessed May 22, 2018.

Pateman, Carol. *Participation and Democratic Theory.* Cambridge: Cambridge University Press, 1970.

Patient-Centered Outcomes Research Institute. "Can CER Help Answer Questions about Hepatitis C? A PCORI Stakeholder Workshop." May 18, 2016. https://www.pcori.org/events/2016/can-cer-help-answer-questions -about-hepatitis-c-pcori-stakeholder-workshop; accessed May 22, 2018.

Patient Protection and Affordable Care Act. 42 U.S.C. § 18001, 2010.

Patients for Stem Cells. http://patientsforstemcells.org/; accessed May 22, 2018.

Pazdur, Richard. "Memorandum to the File BLA 125085 Avastin (bevacizumab): Regulatory Decision to Withdraw Avastin (bevacizumab) Firstline Metastatic Breast Cancer Indication." FDA Center for Drug Evaluation and Research. 2010. https://www.fda.gov/downloads/Drugs/DrugSafety

/PostmarketDrugSafetyInformationforPatientsandProviders/UCM237171
.pdf; accessed May 22, 2018.

Peterson, J. C. and G. E. Markle. "Politics and Science in the Laetrile Controversy." *Social Studies of Science* 9 (1979): 139–66.

Pierson, Paul. "When Effect Becomes Cause: Policy Feedback and Political
Change." *World Politics* 45, no. 04 (1993): 595–628.

Platt, R., N. E. Kass, and D. McGraw. "Ethics, Regulation, and Comparative
Effectiveness Research. Time for Change." *Journal of the American Medical
Association* 311, no. 15 (2014): 1497–98.

Pollack, Andrew. "Breast Cancer Patients Plead for Avastin Approval." *New York
Times.* June 28, 2011. http://www.nytimes.com/2011/06/29/business
/29drug.html; accessed May 22, 2018.

Popp, Berman Elizabeth. "Not Just Neoliberalism: Economization in U.S. Science and Technology Policy." *Science, Technology & Human Values* 39,
no. 3 (2014): 397–431.

Potter, Wendell. "Does the U.S. Have the World's Best Health Care System? Yes,
If You're Talking About the Third World." *Huffington Post.* November 28,
2011. https://www.huffingtonpost.com/wendell-potter/does-the-us-have
-the-best_b_1116105.html; accessed May 22, 2018.

Prasad, Vinay. "Perspective: The Precision-Oncology Illusion." *Nature* 537, no.
7619 (2016): S63.

Prasad, Vinay and Sham Mailankody. "The Accelerated Approval of Oncologic
Drugs: Lessons from Ponatinib." *Journal of the American Medical Association* 311, no. 4 (2014): 353–54.

Prasad, Vinay and A. Vandross. "Characteristics of Exceptional or Super
Responders to Cancer Drugs." *Mayo Clinic Proceedings* 90, no. 12 (2015):
1639–49.

Proust, Marcel. *Swann's Way.* Mineola, NY: Dover Publications, Inc., 2002.

Public Citizen. "RE: Proposed Decision Memo for Beta Amyloid Positron Emission Tomography in Dementia and Neurodegenerative Disease (CAG-
0043IN)." July 23, 2013.

Public Citizen. "Rx R&D Myths: The Case Against the Drug Industry's R&D
'Scare Card.'" *Congress Watch.* July 2001. https://www.citizen.org/sites
/default/files/rdmyths.pdf; accessed May 22, 2018.

Pure Food and Drug Act of 1906. Public Law 59-384.

Quanstrum, Kerianne H. and Rodney A. Hayward. "Lessons from the Mammography Wars." *New England Journal of Medicine* 363, no. 11 (2010):
1076–79.

Rachul, Christen. "'What Have I Got to Lose?' An Analysis of Stem Cell Therapy
Patients' Blogs." *Health Law Review* 20, no. 1 (2011): 5–12.

Ramshaw, Emily. "Perry's Surgery Included Experimental Stem Cell Therapy."
Texas Tribune. August 3, 2011. https://www.texastribune.org/2011/08/03
/perrys-surgery-included-experimental-stem-cell-the/; accessed May 22,
2018.

Reck, M., J. von Pawel, P. Zatloukal, R. Ramlau, V. Gorbounova, V. Hirsh, N. Leigh, J. Mezger, V. Archer, N. Moore, C. Manegold, and the BO17704 Study Group. "Overall Survival with Cisplatin–Gemcitabine and Bevacizumab or Placebo as First-Line Therapy for Nonsquamous Non-Small-Cell Lung Cancer: Results from a Randomised Phase III Trial (AVAiL)." *Annals of Oncology* 21, no. 9 (2010): 1804–09.

Reichard, John. "Baucus, Conrad Offer Bill Creating Comparative Effectiveness Institute." Washington Health Policy Week in Review. August 4, 2008. http://www.commonwealthfund.org/publications/newsletters/washington -health-policy-in-review/2008/aug/washington-health-policy-week-in -review-august-4-2008/baucus-conrad-offer-bill-creating-comparative -effectiveness-institute; accessed May 22, 2018.

Reinhardt. Uwe E. "Divide et Impera: Protecting the Growth of Health Care Incomes (COSTS)." *Health Economics* 21 (2012): 41–54.

Reinhardt, Uwe E. "Probing Our Moral Values in Health Care: The Pricing of Specialty Drugs." *Journal of the American Medical Association* 314, no. 10 (2015): 981–82.

Reinhardt, Uwe E. "The Uproar Over Mammography." Economix, Explaining the Science of Everyday Life. *The New York Times.* November 20, 2009.

Rettig, Richard A., Peter D. Jacobson, Cynthia M. Farquhar, and Wade M. Aubry. *False Hope: Bone Marrow Transplantation for Breast Cancer.* New York: Oxford University Press, 2007.

Reuters Staff. "FDA Approves Gilead's Breakthrough Hepatitis C Pill." Reuters, December 6, 2013. https://www.reuters.com/article/us-gilead-fda-hepatitis /fda-approves-gileads-breakthrough-hepatitis-c-pill-idUSBRE9B50 YB20131206; accessed May 22, 2018.

Richardson, Elizabeth. "Aligning FDA and CMS Review." *Health Affairs Policy Brief.* August 27, 2015. doi: 10.1377/hpb20150827.132391. https://www .healthaffairs.org/do/10.1377/hpb20150827.132391/full/; accessed May 22, 2018.

Richardson, Elizabeth, Joan H. Krause, Jordan Paradise, Rob Lott, and Tracy Gnadinger. "Right-to-Try Laws." Health Policy Brief. *Health Affairs.* April 9, 2015. http://www.healthaffairs.org/healthpolicybriefs/brief.php? brief_id=135; accessed May 22, 2018.

Robinson, James C. "Applying Value-Based Insurance Design to High-Cost Health Services." *Health Affairs* 29, no. 11 (2010): 2009–16.

Rodwin, Mark A. "The Politics of Evidence-Based Medicine." *Journal of Health Politics, Policy, and Law* 26, no. 2 (2011): 438–46.

Ross, Casey. "This Federal Agency that Aims to Make Health Care More Effective Is on the Chopping Block, Again." STAT. March 30, 2017. https://www .statnews.com/2017/03/30/ahrq-budget-trump-nih/; accessed May 22, 2018.

Rowe, G. and L.J. Frewer. "A Typology of Public Engagement Mechanisms." *Science, Technology & Human Values* 30, no. 2 (2005): 25–90.

Rutter, K., A. F. Stättermayer, S. Beinhardt, T. M. Scherzer, P. Steindl-Munda, and M. Trauner. "Successful Antiviral Treatment Improves Survival of Patients with Advanced Liver Disease Due to Chronic Hepatitis C." *Aliment Pharmacology Therapy* 41 (2015): 521–31.

Saltz, Leonard B. "Can Money Really Be No Object When Cancer Care Is the Subject?" *Journal of Clinical Oncology* 33, no. 10 (2015): 1093–94.

Salzman, Sony. "How Insurance Providers Deny Hepatitis C Patients Lifesaving Drugs." *Al Jazeera America.* October 19, 2015. http://america.aljazeera .com/articles/2015/10/16/insurance-providers-deny-hepatitis-drugs .html; accessed May 22, 2018.

Sanders, Bernard. "Opening Statement. Hepatitis C and Veterans." Hearing before the Committee on Veterans' Affairs, One Hundred Thirteenth Congress, Second Session. December 3, 2014.

Sarkar, Souvik, Zhen Jiang, Donna M. Evon, Abdus S. Wahed, and Jay H. Hoofnagle. "Fatigue Before, During, and after Antiviral Therapy of Chronic Hepatitis C: Results from the Virahep-C Study." *Journal of Hepatology* 57 (2012): 946–52.

Scharf, Amy and Elizabeth Dzeng. "'I'm Willing to Try Anything': Compassionate Use Access to Experimental Drugs and the Misguided Mission of Right-to -Try Laws." *Health Affairs Blog.* March 27, 2017. https://www.healthaffairs .org/do/10.1377/hblog20170327.059378/full/; accessed May 22, 2018.

Schelling, Thomas C. "The Life You Save May Be Your Own." In *Problems in Public Expenditure Analysis*, edited by S. B. Chaase, 127–76. Washington, D.C.: The Brookings Institution, 1968.

Schiff, L. "Finding Truth in a World Full of Spin: Myth-Busting in the Case of Sovaldi." *Clinical Therapeutics* 37, no. 5 (2015): 1092–1112.

Schneider, Anne and Helen Ingram. "Social Construction of Target Populations: Implications for Politics and Policy." *American Political Science Review* 87, no. 2 (1993): 3343–47.

Schön, D. and M. Rein. *Frame Reflection: Toward the Resolution of Intractable Policy Controversies*. New York: Basic Books, 1994.

Schulte, Fred. "Is Obamacare's Research Institute Worth the Billions?" NPR. August 4, 2015. http://www.npr.org/sections/health-shots/2015/08/04 /428164731/is-obamacares-research-institute-worth-the-billions; accessed May 22, 2018.

Servick, Kelly. "'Right to Try' Laws Bypass FDA for Last-ditch Treatments." *Science* 344, no. 6190 (2014): 1329.

Servick, Kelly. "Texas Has Sanctioned Unapproved Stem Cell Therapies. Will It Change Anything?" *Science.* June 15, 2017. http://www.sciencemag.org /news/2017/06/texas-has-sanctioned-unapproved-stem-cell-therapies-will -it-change-anything; H.B. 810. http://www.capitol.state.tx.us/tlodocs/85R /billtext/pdf/HB00810E.pdf#navpanes=0; accessed May 22, 2018.

Shapiro, Jeffrey K. "FDA to Hold a Public Hearing for a Quartet of Draft HCT/P Guidances: A Scorecard." FDA Law Blog. November 2, 2015. http://www

.fdalawblog.net/2015/11/fda-to-hold-a-public-hearing-for-a-quartet-of -draft-hctp-guidances-a-scorecard/; accessed May 22, 2018.

Shewhart, W. A. *Statistical Method from the Viewpoint of Quality Control.* Mineola, NY: Dover Publications, 1986.

Shih, T. and C. Lindley. "Bevacizumab: An Angiogenesis Inhibitor for the Treatment of Solid Malignancies." *Clinical Therapeutics* 28, no. 11 (2006): 1779–1802.

Siegel, Michael. "Don't Let Alternative Facts Deter Congress From Fixing e-cigarette Regulations." *Washington Examiner.* May 2, 2017. http://www.washingtonex-aminer.com/dont-let-alternative-facts-deter-congress-from-fixing-e -cigarette-regulations/article/262182; accessed May 22, 2018.

Sifferlin, Alexandra. "Breast Cancer Screening: How Komen Oversold the Bene-fits of Mammography." *Time.* August 3, 2012. http://healthland.time .com/2012/08/03/breast-cancer-screening-komen-ad-overstated-the -benefits-of-mammography-researchers-say/; accessed May 22, 2018.

Silverman, E. "Avastin & FDA Were Both on Trial: Dan Explains." *Pharmalot. com.* June 20, 2011. http://pharmalot.com/2011/06/avastin-fda-were -both-on-trial-carpenter-explains/; accessed May 22, 2018.

Silverman, E. "Lilly Backs Lawsuit Against CMS Over Its Alzheimer's Diagnostic Drug." *Wall Street Journal.* September 5, 2014. http://blogs.wsj.com /pharmalot/2014/09/05/lilly-backs-lawsuit-against-cms-over-its -alzheimers-diagnostic-drug/; accessed May 22, 2018.

Singal, Amit G., Michael L. Volk, Donald Jensen, Adrian M. Di Bisceglie, and Philip S. Schoenfeld. "A Sustained Viral Response Ys Associated with Reduced Liver-Related Morbidity and Mortality in Patients with Hepatitis C Virus." *Clinical Gastroenterology and Hepatology* 8 (2010): 280–88, 288.e1.

Singh, Gopal K. and Ahmedin Jemal. "Socioeconomic and Racial/Ethnic Dis-parities in Cancer Mortality, Incidence, and Survival in the United States, 1950–2014: Over Six Decades of Changing Patterns and Widening Inequalities." *Journal of Environmental and Public Health* (2017). https:// doi.org/10.1155/2017/2819372; https://www.hindawi.com/journals/jeph /2017/2819372/abs/; accessed May 22, 2018.

Skocpol, Theda. *Protecting Soldiers and Mothers: The Political Origins of Social Policy in the United States.* Cambridge, MA: Belknap Press of Harvard University Press, 1992.

Sledge, George W., Eleftherios P. Mamounas, Gabriel N. Hortobagyi, Harold J. Burstein, Pamela J. Goodwin, and Antonio C. Wolff. "Past, Present, and Future Challenges in Breast Cancer Treatment." *Journal of Clinical Oncol-ogy* 32, no. 19 (2014): 1979–86.

Smith v. Burwell. No. 14-1519. U.S. District Court for the District of Columbia, December 12, 2014.

Social Security Act Sec. 1862, 42 U.S.C. 1395y (a) (1)(A).

Solomon, M. Z., M. K. Gusmano, and K. J. Maschke. "The Ethical Imperative and Moral Challenges of Engaging Patients and the Public with Evi-dence." *Health Affairs* 35 (2015): 4583–89.

Solomon, Miriam. *Making Medical Knowledge.* Oxford: Oxford University Press, 2015.

Solomon, Stephanie and Julia Abelson. "Why and When Should We Use Public Deliberation?" *Hastings Center Report* 42, no. 2 (2012): 17–20.

Sorenson, C., M. K. Gusmano, and A. Oliver. "The Politics of Comparative-Effectiveness Research: Lessons from Recent History." *Journal of Health Politics, Policy and Law* 3, no. 1 (2014): 139–69.

Starr, Paul. *Remedy and Reaction: The Peculiar American Struggle over Health Care Reform,* Revised edition. New Haven, CT: Yale University Press, 2013.

Starr, Paul. *The Social Transformation of American Medicine: The Rise of a Sovereign Profession and the Making of a Vast Industry.* New York: Basic Books, 1982.

Staton, Tracy. "Gilead and Express Scripts Make Peace in Hep C with 2017 Formulary Deal." FiercePharma. December 15, 2016. https://www.fiercepharma.com/pharma/gilead-and-express-scripts-make-peace-hep-c-2017-formulary-deal; accessed May 22, 2018.

Stein, Rob. "FDA Considers Revoking Approval of Avastin for Advanced Breast Cancer." *Washington Post.* August 16, 2010. http://www.washingtonpost.com/wp-dyn/content/article/2010/08/15/AR2010081503466.html; accessed May 22, 2018.

Stein, Sam, Ryan Grim, and Matt Fuller. "Congress Is About to Pass a Bill That Shows D.C. at Its Worst—It May Also Turn Around the Opioid Crisis and Cure Cancer." *Huffington Post.* November 29, 2016. https://www.huffingtonpost.com/entry/congress-21st-century-cures_us_583e3d98e4b0ae0e7cdaca32; accessed May 22, 2018.

Steinbrook, Robert. "The Centers for Medicare & Medicaid Services and Amyloid-β Positron Emission Tomography for Alzheimer Disease." *Journal of the American Medical Association Internal Medicine* 174, no. 1 (2014): 135.

Stevens, Rosemary. *The Public-Private Health Care State: Essays on the History of American Health Care Policy.* New Brunswick, NJ: Transaction Publishers, 2007.

Strach, Patricia. *Hiding Politics in Plain Sight: Cause Marketing, Corporate Influence, and Breast Cancer Policymaking.* New York: Oxford University Press, 2016.

Sur, Roger L. and Philipp Dahm. "History of Evidence-Based Medicine." *Indian Journal of Urology* 27, no. 4 (2011): 487–89.

"Susan G. Komen for the Cure® Scientific Advisory Board's Perspective on the U.S. Preventive Service Task Force (USPSTF) Recommendations on Breast Screening." November 2009. https://ww5.komen.org/ResearchAndGrants/PerspectiveOnUSPSTFRecommendationsOnScreening.aspx; accessed May 22, 2018.

Swetlitz, Ike. "In State of Union, Trump Endorses 'Right to Try' For Terminally Ill Patients." STAT. January 30, 2018. https://www.statnews.com/2018/01/30/state-of-the-union-trump-right-to-try/; accessed May 22, 2018.

Szabo, Liz. "Breakthrough Cancer Drug Could Be Astronomical in Price." *USA Today.* August 22, 2017. https://www.usatoday.com/story/news/2017

/08/22/breakthrough-cancer-drug-astronomical-price/589442001/; accessed May 22, 2018.

Szabo, Liz. "Cascade of Costs Could Push New Gene Therapy Above $1 Million Per Patient." *Kaiser Health News*. October 17, 2017. https://khn.org/news /cascade-of-costs-could-push-new-gene-therapy-above-1-million-per -patient/; accessed May 22, 2018.

Tanne, Janice Hopkins. "Celebrity Illnesses Raise Awareness, but Can Give Wrong Message." *BMJ* 321 no. 7369 (2000): 1099.

Tannenbaum, Sandra J. "Particularism in Health Care: Challenging the Author- ity of the Aggregate." *Journal of Evaluation in Clinical Practice* 20 (2014): 934–41.

Thomas, Archibald. "They Just Know: The Epistemological Politics of 'Evidence- Based' Non-Formal Education." *Evaluation and Program Planning* 48 (2015): 137–48.

Thomas, Katie. "Insurers Battle Families Over Costly Drug for Fatal Disease." *New York Times*. June 22, 2017. https://www.nytimes.com/2017/06/22 /health/duchenne-muscular-dystrophy-drug-exondys-51.html; accessed May 22, 2018.

Thomas, Katie. "Trump Vows to Ease Rules for Drug Makers, but Again Zeros in on Prices." *New York Times*. January 31, 2017. https://www.nytimes .com/2017/01/31/health/trump-vows-to-ease-rules-for-drug-makers -but-prices-remain-a-focus.html; accessed May 22, 2018.

Thomas, Katie. "Trump's F.D.A. Pick Could Undo Decades of Drug Safeguards." *New York Times*. February 5, 2017. https://www.nytimes.com/2017/02/05 /health/with-fda-vacancy-trump-sees-chance-to-speed-drugs-to-the -market.html.

Timmermans, Stefan and Marc Berg. *The Gold Standard: The Challenge of Evidence- Based Medicine and Standardization in Health Care*. Philadelphia: Temple University Press, 2010.

Toich, Laurie. "Will Hepatitis C Virus Medication Costs Drop in the Years Ahead?" *Pharmacy Times*. February 8, 2017. http://www.pharmacytimes .com/resource-centers/hepatitisc/will-hepatitis-c-virus-medicaton-costs -drop-in-the-years-ahead; accessed May 22, 2018.

Trickett, Wendler, Frank Mongiello, Jordan McLinn, and Matthew Bellina. "Right to Try Act of 2017." https://www.congress.gov/bill/115th-congress /senate-bill/204; accessed May 22, 2018.

Trooskin, Stacey B., Helen Reynolds, and Jay R. Kostman. "Access to Costly New Hepatitis C Drugs: Medicine, Money, and Advocacy." *Clinical Infectious Diseases* 61, no. 2 (2015): 1825–30.

Trosman, J. R., S. L. Van Bebber, and K. A. Phillips. "Coverage Policy Development for Personalized Medicine: Private Payer Perspectives on Developing Policy for the 21-Gene Assay." *Journal of Oncology Practice* 6, no. 5 (2010): 238–42.

Trosman, J. R., S. L. Van Bebber, and K. A. Phillips. "Health Technology Assess- ment and Private Payers' Coverage of Personalized Medicine." *Journal of Oncology Practice* 7, no. 3S (2011): 18s–24s.

Trosman, J. R., C. B. Weldon, R. K. Kelley, and K. A. Phillips. "Challenges of Coverage Policy Development for Next-Generation Tumor Sequencing Panels: Experts and Payers Weigh In." *Journal of the National Comprehensive Cancer Network* 13, no. 3 (2015): 312–18.

Trosman, J. R., C. B. Weldon, J. C. Schink, W. J. Gradishar, and A. B. Benson. "What Do Providers, Payers, and Patients Need from Comparative -Effectiveness Research on Diagnostics? The Case of HER2/Neu Testing in Breast Cancer." *Journal of Comparative Effectiveness Research* 2, no. 4 (2013): 461–77.

Truman, David. *The Government Process: Political Interests and Public Opinion.* New York: Alfred A. Knopf, 1951.

Trump, Donald J. "President Donald J. Trump's State of the Union Address." The White House. January 30, 2018. https://www.whitehouse.gov/briefings -statements/president-donald-j-trumps-state-union-address/; accessed May 22, 2018.

Tuckson, Reed and Daniel S. Blumenthal. "Why Aren't Millions of Americans Getting Preventive Care?" STAT. April 15, 2016. https://www.statnews .com/2016/04/15/preventive-care-public-health/; accessed May 22, 2018.

Turner, Leigh. "US Stem Cell Clinics, Patient Safety, and the FDA." *Trends in Molecular Medicine* 21, no. 5 (2015): 271–73.

Turner, Leigh and Paul Knoepfler. "Selling Stem Cells in the USA: Assessing the Direct-to-Consumer Industry." *Cell Stem Cell* 19, no. 2 (2016): 154–57.

Twenty-First Century Cures Act. http://docs.house.gov/billsthisweek/20161128 /CPRT-114-HPRT-RU00-SAHR34.pdf; accessed May 22, 2018.

UNAIDS. "90-90-90: An Ambitious Treatment Target to Help End the AIDS Epidemic." Joint United Nations Programme on HIV/AIDS (UNAIDS). October 2014.

UPI. "Sebelius: Mammogram Policies Unchanged." *UPI Top News.* November 18, 2009. https://www.upi.com/Top_News/US/2009/11/18/Sebelius -Mammogram-policies-unchanged/UPI-18271258591793/; accessed May 22, 2018.

U.S. Senate. *Mammography: Hearings before a Subcommittee of the Committee on Appropriations.* United States Senate, One Hundred Fifth Congress, First Session. Special Hearings. Washington, D.C.: Government Printing Office, 1997. https://www.gpo.gov/fdsys/pkg/CHRG-105shrg44044 /html/CHRG-105shrg44044.htm; accessed May 22, 2018.

U.S. Senate. REGROW Act. 114th Congress. https://www.congress.gov /bill/114th-congress/senate-bill/2689; accessed May 22, 2018.

U.S. v. Regenerative Sciences, Civ. Action No. 10-1327 (RMC). Memorandum Opinion, July 23, 2012.

U.S. v. Regenerative Sciences, 848 F. Supp. 2d 248 (2012).

van der Meer, A. J., Bart J. Veldt, Jordan J. Feld, Heiner Wedemeyer, Jean-François Dufour, Frank Lammert, Andrés Duarte-Rojo, Elizabeth Jenny Heathcote, Michael P. Manns, Lorenz Kuske, Stefan Zeuzem, W. Peter Hofmann, Robert Jacobus de Knegt, Bettina E. Hansen, and Harry L. A. Janssen.

"Association Between Sustained Virological Response and All-Cause Mortality Among Patients with Chronic Hepatitis C and Advanced Hepatic Fibrosis." *Journal of the American Medical Association* 308 (2010): 2584–93.

Vitry, A., T. Nguyen, V. Entwistle, and E. Roughead. "Regulatory Withdrawal of Medicines Marketed with Uncertain Benefits: The Bevacizumab Case Study." *Journal of Pharmaceutical Policy and Practice* 8 (2015): 25.

Vladeck, Bruce C., Emily J. Goodwin, Lois P. Myers, and Madeline Sinisi. "Consumers and Hospital Use: The HCFA 'Death List.'" *Health Affairs* 7, no. 1 (1988): 122–25.

Vladeck, Bruce C. and Thomas Rice. "Market Failure and the Failure of Discourse: Facing Up to the Power of Sellers." *Health Affairs* 28, no. 5 (2009): 1305–15.

von Eschenbach, Andrew. "Medical Innovation: How the U.S. Can Retain Its Lead," *Wall Street Journal.* February 14, 2012. https://www.wsj.com/articles/SB10001424052970203646004577215403399350874; accessed May 22, 2018.

Wall Street Journal. "Liberals and Mammography: Rationing? What Rationing?" Review and Outlook. *The Wall Street Journal* Online. November 24, 2009. https://www.wsj.com/articles/SB10001424052748704779704574552320 222125990; accessed May 22, 2018.

Wehrle, Edmund F. "For a Healthy America." *Labor's Heritage* 28, Summer (1993): 40.

Weintraub, Arlene. "How to Cover Novartis' $475K CAR-T Drug Kymriah? A 'New Payment Model' Is the Only Way, Express Scripts Says." FiercePharma. September 22, 2017. https://www.fiercepharma.com/financials/car-t-and-other-gene-therapies-need-new-payment-model-says-express-scripts; accessed May 22, 2018.

Weir, Margaret, Ann Shola Orloff, and Theda Skocpol. *The Politics of Social Policy in the United States.* Princeton, NJ: Princeton University Press, 1988.

Weissman, Irving. "Stem Cell Therapies Could Change Medicine . . . If They Get the Chance." *Cell Stem Cell* 10 (2012): 663–65.

Wells, Jane. "Mammography Screening and the Politics of Randomised Trials." *BMJ* 317, no. 7172 (1998): 1224–30.

Wennberg, John. "AHCPR and the Strategy for Health Care Reform." *Health Affairs* 11, no. 4 (1992): 67–72.

Wennberg, John. "Forty Years of Unwarranted Variation—And Still Counting." *Health Policy* 114 (2014): 1–2.

Wennberg, John. "The More Things Change . . . The Federal Government's Role in Evaluative Sciences." *Health Affairs* 2003: W3-308–10.

Wennberg, John and A. Gittelsohn. "Small Area Variations in Health Care Delivery: A Population-Based Health Information System Can Guide Planning and Regulatory Decision-Making." *Science* 182, no. 4117 (1973): 110211–08.

White, Joseph. "Prices, Volume, and the Perverse Effects of the Variations Crusade." *Journal of Health Politics, Policy and Law* 36, no. 4 (2011): 775–90.

White, Kerr L., T. Franklin Williams, and Bernard G. Greenberg. "The Ecology of Medical Care. 1961." *Bulletin of the New York Academy of Medicine* 73, no. 1 (1996): 187.

Wilcken, Nicholas. "How Breast Cancer Treatment Has Evolved Since the 1950s." *American Council on Society and Health*. June 1, 2016. https://www.acsh.org/news/2016/06/01/how-breast-cancer-treatment-has-evolved-since-the-1950s; accessed May 22, 2018.

Wildavsky, Aaron. "Doing Better and Feeling Worse: The Political Pathology of Health Policy." In *The Art and Craft of Policy Analysis*. London: Palgrave Macmillan, 1979.

Wilensky, Gail R. "Developing a Center for Comparative Effectiveness Information." *Health Affairs* 25, no. 6 (2006): w572–w585.

Wilensky, Gail R. "The Mammography Guidelines and Evidence-Based Medicine." *Health Affairs Blog*, January 12, 2010. https://www.healthaffairs.org/do/10.1377/hblog20100112.003427/full/; accessed May 22, 2018.

Wilkinson, Richard and Michael Marmot, eds. *The Solid Facts*, 2nd edition. Copenhagen: The World Health Organization, 1999.

Williams, David. "ObamaCare Demonstrates Dangers of Government Interference." *The Hill*. November 2, 2016. http://origin-nyi.thehill.com/blogs/pundits-blog/healthcare/304066-obamacare-demonstrates-dangers-of-government-interference; accessed May 22, 2018.

Woloshin, S., L. M. Schwartz, W. C. Black, and B. S. Kramer. "Cancer Screening Campaigns—Getting Past Uninformative Persuasion." *New England Journal of Medicine* 367, no. 18 (2012): 1677–79.

Woolf, Steven H., Corinne G. Husten, Lawrence S. Lewin, James S. Marks, Jonathan E. Fielding, and Eduardo J. Sanchez. *The Economic Argument for Disease Prevention: Distinguishing Between Value and Savings.* A Prevention Policy Paper Commissioned by Partnership for Prevention, 2009.

Woolley, J. Patrick. "Kaufman's Debt to Kant: The Epistemological Importance of the 'Structure of the World Which Environs Us.'" *Zygon* 48, no. 3 (2013): 544–64.

Wright, Tiffany C. "The Average Profit Margin of Pharmaceuticals." May 22, 2018. *azcentral.com*. https://yourbusiness.azcentral.com/average-profit-margin-pharmaceuticals-20671.html; accessed June 12, 2018.

Wulff, Katherine Cooper, Franklin G. Miller, and Steven D. Pearson. "Can Coverage Be Rescinded When Negative Trial Results Threaten a Popular Procedure? The Ongoing Saga of Vertebroplasty." *Health Affairs* 30, no. 12 (2011): 2269–76.

Index

About the Authors

Karen J. Maschke, PhD, is a research scholar at The Hastings Center, a bioethics research institute in Garrison, New York. She has a PhD in political science from Johns Hopkins University and a master's degree in bioethics from Case Western Reserve University. Prior to joining The Hastings Center, she was a college professor, teaching a wide range of courses related to American government and politics, law and society, and constitutional law. Dr. Maschke has expertise on the ethical, legal, and policy issues associated with new biomedical technologies. She has published three previous books, including (as coeditor) *Performance-Enhancing Technologies in Sports: Ethical, Conceptual, and Scientific Issues* (2009). She is currently the editor of *IRB: Ethics & Human Research*.

Michael K. Gusmano, PhD, is an associate professor of health systems and policy at the Rutgers University School of Public Health, a research scholar at The Hastings Center, and a visiting fellow at the Rockefeller Institute of Government, SUNY. He has a PhD from the University of Maryland at College Park and was a postdoctoral fellow in the Robert Wood Johnson Foundation Scholars in Health Policy Program at Yale University. Dr. Gusmano's research focuses on health system reform and comparative health policy. His research interests include questions about access to health care for poor and other vulnerable groups and the regulation of technology. He has published five previous books and more than 100 scholarly articles and essays and is currently an associate editor for the *Journal of Aging and Social Policy* and *Health Economics, Policy, and Law*.